Hysterectomy and the Alternatives

Editors

JOHN A. OCCHINO
EMANUEL C. TRABUCO

OBSTETRICS AND GYNECOLOGY CLINICS OF NORTH AMERICA

www.obgyn.theclinics.com

Consulting Editor
WILLIAM F. RAYBURN

September 2016 • Volume 43 • Number 3

ELSEVIER

1600 John F. Kennedy Boulevard • Suite 1800 • Philadelphia, Pennsylvania, 19103-2899

http://www.theclinics.com

OBSTETRICS AND GYNECOLOGY CLINICS OF NORTH AMERICA Volume 43, Number 3
September 2016 ISSN 0889-8545, ISBN-13: 978-0-323-46262-4

Editor: Kerry Holland
Developmental Editor: Kristen Helm

Obstetrics and Gynecology Clinics (ISSN 0889-8545) is published quarterly by Elsevier Inc., 360 Park Avenue South, New York, NY 10010-1710. Months of issue are March, June, September, and December. Periodicals postage paid at New York, NY, and additional mailing offices. Subscription price per year is $295.00 (US individuals), $597.00 (US institutions), $100.00 (US students), $370.00 (Canadian individuals), $754.00 (Canadian institutions), $225.00 (Canadian students), $450.00 (international individuals), $754.00 (international institutions), and $225.00 (international students). To receive student/resident rate, orders must be accompanied by name of affiliated institution, date of term, and the signature of program/residency coordinator on institution letterhead. Orders will be billed at individual rate until proof of status is received. Foreign air speed delivery is included in all *Clinics* subscription prices. All prices are subject to change without notice. POSTMASTER: Send address changes to *Obstetrics and Gynecology Clinics*, Elsevier Health Sciences Division, Subscription Customer Service, 3251 Riverport Lane, Maryland Heights, MO 63043. **Customer Service: Telephone: 1-800-654-2452 (U.S. and Canada); 314-447-8871 (outside U.S. and Canada). Fax: 314-447-8029. E-mail: journalscustomerservice-usa@elsevier.com (for print support); journalsonlinesupport-usa@elsevier. com (for online support).**

Reprints. For copies of 100 or more of articles in this publication, please contact the Commercial Reprints Department, Elsevier Inc., 360 Park Avenue South, New York, New York 10010-1710. Tel.: 212-633-3874; Fax: 212-633-3820; E-mail: reprints@elsevier.com.

Obstetrics and Gynecology Clinics of North America is also published in Spanish by McGraw-Hill Interamericana Editores S.A., P.O. Box 5-237, 06500, Mexico; in Portuguese by Reichmann and Affonso Editores, Rio de Janeiro, Brazil; and in Greek by Paschalidis Medical Publications, Athens, Greece.

Obstetrics and Gynecology Clinics of North America is covered in MEDLINE/PubMed (Index Medicus), Excerpta Medica, Current Concepts/Clinical Medicine, Science Citation Index, BIOSIS, CINAHL, and ISI/BIOMED.

Contributors

CONSULTING EDITOR

WILLIAM F. RAYBURN, MD, MBA
Associate Dean, Continuing Medical Education and Professional Development,
Distinguished Professor and Emeritus Chair, Obstetrics and Gynecology, University of
New Mexico School of Medicine, Albuquerque, New Mexico

EDITORS

JOHN A. OCCHINO, MD, MS
Assistant Professor, Division of Gynecologic Surgery, Department of Obstetrics and
Gynecology, Mayo Clinic, Rochester, Minnesota

EMANUEL C. TRABUCO, MD, MS
Assistant Professor, Division of Gynecologic Surgery, Department of Obstetrics and
Gynecology, Mayo Clinic, Rochester, Minnesota

AUTHORS

ARNOLD P. ADVINCULA, MD, FACOG, FACS
Levine Family Professor of Women's Health; Vice-Chair, Department of Obstetrics and
Gynecology; Chief of Gynecology, Sloane Hospital for Women; Medical Director,
Simulation Center, Columbia University Medical Center, New York-Presbyterian Hospital,
New York, New York

MATTHEW A. BARKER, MD
Associate Professor, Departments of Obstetrics and Gynecology and Internal Medicine,
Sanford School of Medicine, The University of South Dakota, Vermillion, South Dakota;
Director of Female Pelvic Medicine and Reconstructive Surgery, Avera McKennan
Hospital and University Center, Sioux Falls, South Dakota

MEGAN R. BILLOW, DO
Departments of Obstetrics and Gynecology; Reproductive Biology, University Hospitals,
Case Medical Center, Cleveland, Ohio

ERIN A. BRENNAND, MD
Assistant Professor, Department of Obstetrics and Gynecology, University of Calgary,
Calgary, Alberta, Canada

JENIFER N. BYRNES, DO
Fellow, Female Pelvic Medicine and Reconstructive Surgery, Mayo Clinic, Rochester,
Minnesota

SEAN C. DOWDY, MD
Professor of Obstetrics and Gynecology; Chair, Division of Gynecologic Surgery, Mayo Clinic, Rochester, Minnesota

SHERIF A. EL-NASHAR, MD, PhD
Departments of Obstetrics and Gynecology; Reproductive Biology, University Hospitals, Case Medical Center, Cleveland, Ohio; Department of Obstetrics and Gynecology, Assiut University, Assiut, Egypt

DOBIE GILES, MD, MS
Assistant Professor, Division of Gynecology and Gynecologic Subspecialties, Department of Obstetrics and Gynecology, University of Wisconsin-Madison, Madison, Wisconsin

CHRISTOPHER KEVIN HULS, MD, MSc
Clinical Assistant Professor, Department of Obstetrics and Gynecology, Banner University Medical Center, College of Medicine – Phoenix, University of Arizona; Medical Director, Phoenix Perinatal Associates of Mednax, Inc, Phoenix, Arizona

ELEFTHERIA KALOGERA, MD
Instructor in Obstetrics and Gynecology; Resident Physician, Department of Obstetrics and Gynecology, Mayo Clinic, Rochester, Minnesota

SHUNAHA KIM-FINE, MD, MS
Clinical Assistant Professor, Department of Obstetrics and Gynecology, University of Calgary, Calgary, Alberta, Canada

CARA R. KING, DO, MS
Assistant Professor, Division of Gynecology and Gynecologic Subspecialties, Department of Obstetrics and Gynecology, University of Wisconsin-Madison, Madison, Wisconsin

SHANNON K. LAUGHLIN-TOMMASO, MD, MPH
Assistant Professor, Departments of Obstetrics and Gynecology and Surgery, Mayo Clinic, Rochester, Minnesota

CATHERINE A. MATTHEWS, MD, FACOG, FACS
Professor of Obstetrics and Gynecology and Urology, Wake Forest University Medical Center, Winston Salem, North Carolina

MICHAEL MOEN, MD, FACOG, FACS
Professor, Obstetrics and Gynecology, Chicago Medical School, Rosalind Franklin University, North Chicago, Illinois

JOHN A. OCCHINO, MD, MS
Assistant Professor, Division of Gynecologic Surgery, Department of Obstetrics and Gynecology, Mayo Clinic, Rochester, Minnesota

KHARA M. SIMPSON, MD
Minimally Invasive Gynecologic Surgery Fellow, Gynecologic Specialty Surgery, Department of Obstetrics and Gynecology, Columbia University Medical Center, New York, New York

EMANUEL C. TRABUCO, MD, MS
Assistant Professor, Division of Gynecologic Surgery, Department of Obstetrics and Gynecology, Mayo Clinic, Rochester, Minnesota

Contents

Uterine fibroids are a common condition that can be debilitating and are the leading benign cause of hysterectomy. Women often live with the symptoms rather than choose hysterectomy, but survey studies have shown that work, social life, and physical activities are hindered by fibroid symptoms. Offering alternative therapies tailored to a woman's symptoms will allow her to choose a treatment that fits her needs and to preserve her uterus and fertility. The minimally invasive treatment options have a faster recovery and lower surgical risk than hysterectomy, but may require reintervention. One pharmacologic treatment offers short-term, intermittent therapy with lasting effects.

Abnormal uterine bleeding (AUB) is a common problem that negatively impacts a woman's health-related quality of life and activity. Initial medical treatment includes hormonal and nonhormonal medications. If bleeding persists and no structural abnormalities are present, a repeat trial of medical therapy, a levonorgestrel intrauterine system, or an endometrial ablation can be used dependent on future fertility wishes. The levonorgestrel intrauterine system and endometrial ablation are effective, less invasive, and safe alternatives to a hysterectomy in women with AUB. A hysterectomy is the definitive treatment of AUB irrespective of the suspected cause when alternative treatments fail. Future studies should focus on detection of predictors for treatment outcomes.

Hysterectomy is the most common major gynecologic procedure. Although alternatives to hysterectomy result in fewer procedures performed annually, and the use of endoscopic techniques and vaginal hysterectomy have resulted in a lower percentage performed by the open abdominal route, certain pelvic disorders require abdominal hysterectomy. Preoperative evaluation with informed consent and surgical planning are essential to select appropriate candidates. Prophylactic antibiotics, thromboprophylaxis, attention to surgical technique, and enhanced recovery protocols should be used to provide optimal outcomes.

As minimally invasive technology continues to be developed and refined, surgeons must be discerning in choosing the safest, cost-effective surgical approach associated with the best outcomes for each individual patient. Vaginal hysterectomy can be successfully accomplished even in challenging situations, such as previous pelvic surgery, nulliparity, uterine enlargement, or obesity. Vaginal hysterectomy should be considered the primary route for treatment of benign disease.

Vaginal hysterectomy has been shown to have the lowest complication rate, better cosmesis, and decreased cost compared with alternate routes of hysterectomy. However, there are times when a vaginal hysterectomy is not feasible and an open abdominal hysterectomy should be avoided. Minimally invasive surgery has evolved over the last several decades; with the improvement in optics and surgical instruments, laparoscopic hysterectomy is becoming increasingly common. A total laparoscopic hysterectomy is possible with proper training, including sound technique in laparoscopic suturing for closure of the vaginal cuff.

 Video content accompanies this article at http://www.obgyn. theclinics.com.

Robotic-assisted laparoscopic hysterectomies are being performed at higher rates since the da Vinci Surgical System (Intuitive Surgical, Inc, Sunnyvale, CA, USA) received US Food and Drug Administration approval in 2005 for gynecologic procedures. Despite the technological advancements over traditional laparoscopy, a discrepancy exists between what the literature states and what the benefits are as seen through the eyes of the end-user. There remains a significant learning curve in the adoption of safe and efficient robotic skills. The authors present important considerations when choosing to perform a robotic hysterectomy and a step-by-step technique. The literature on perioperative outcomes is also reviewed.

Although vaginal hysterectomy has long been championed by the American College of Obstetricians and Gynecologists as the preferred mode of uterine removal, nationwide vaginal hysterectomy utilization has steadily declined. This article reviews the evidence comparing vaginal with other modes of hysterectomy and highlights areas of ongoing controversy regarding contraindications to vaginal surgery, risk of subsequent prolapse development, and impacts of changing hysterectomy trends on resident education.

Hysterectomy at the time of an obstetric delivery or postpartum is an uncommon time to perform one of the most common gynecologic procedures. Hysterectomy associated with pregnancy is often unplanned and undesired. Postpartum complications associated with the need for hysterectomy carry significant risks, which pose challenges for mother-infant bonding and can signify an unexpected end to fertility. The most common indication for hysterectomy is postpartum hemorrhage. Postpartum hemorrhage is caused by uterine atony, genital tract laceration, uterine rupture, invasive placentation, infection, or coagulopathy. Multidisciplinary teams improve outcomes and are capable of managing complex medical and surgical complications that occur postpartum.

Gynecologists performing hysterectomy for benign disease must universally counsel women about ovarian management. The beneficial effect of elective bilateral salpingo-oophorectomy (BSO) on incident ovarian and breast cancer and elimination of need for subsequent adnexal surgery must be weighed against the risks of ovarian hormone withdrawal. Ovarian conservation rates have increased significantly over the past 15 years. In postmenopausal women, however, BSO can reduce ovarian and breast cancer rates without an adverse impact on coronary heart disease, sexual dysfunction, hip fractures, or cognitive function.

A paucity of data exists regarding traditional perioperative practices (bowel preparation, NPO at midnight, liberal narcotics, PCA use, liberal fluids, prolonged bowel and bed rest). Enhanced Recovery after Surgery (ERAS) is an evidence-based approach to peri-operative care associated with improved outcomes including earlier return of gastrointestinal function, reduced opioid use, shorter hospital stay, and substantial cost reductions with stable complication and readmission rates. Basic principles include patient education, minimizing preoperative fasting, avoiding bowel preparation, preemptive analgesia, nausea/vomiting prophylaxis, perioperative euvolemia, no routine use of drain and nasogastric tubes, early mobilization, oral intake, and catheter removal, non-opioid analgesics, and preemptive laxatives.

Simulation in surgical training is playing an increasingly important role as postgraduate medical education programs navigate an environment of increasing costs of education, increased attention on patient safety, and new duty hour restrictions. In obstetrics and gynecology, simulation has been used to teach many procedures; however, it lacks a standardized curriculum. Several different simulators exist for teaching various routes and aspects of hysterectomy. This article describes how a formal framework of increasing levels of competencies can be applied to simulation in teaching the procedure of hysterectomy.

Hysterectomy is one of the most common gynecologic surgeries. Early adoption of surgical advancements in hysterectomies has raised concerns over safety, quality, and costs. The risk of potential leiomyosarcoma in women undergoing minimally invasive hysterectomy led the US Food and Drug Administration to discourage the use of electronic power morcellator. Minimally invasive hysterectomies have increased substantially despite lack of data supporting its use over other forms of hysterectomy and increased costs. Health care reform is incentivizing providers to improve quality, improve safety, and decrease costs through standardized outcomes and process measures.

OBSTETRICS AND GYNECOLOGY CLINICS

THE CLINICS ARE AVAILABLE ONLINE!
Access your subscription at:
www.theclinics.com

Foreword

Fewer Hysterectomies and So Many Alternatives

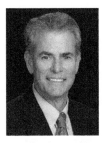

William F. Rayburn, MD, MBA
Consulting Editor

This issue of *Obstetrics and Gynecology Clinics of North America* tackles the very relevant subject, "Hysterectomy and the Alternatives." Being well organized by the guest editors, Dr John Occhino and Dr Emanuel Trabuco, this issue highlights how hysterectomy remains one of the most commonly performed surgical procedures in women despite a national trend that it is being performed less. Estimates suggest that one in nine women will undergo a hysterectomy during their lifetime. This ratio is declining at a time when the number of adult women in the United States is increasing.

The editors chose an expert group of authors, who provided their insights into topics that have a strong influence on the practice of gynecologic surgery. Although a hysterectomy is the treatment for most women with gynecologic malignancies, uterine-sparing treatment is now often used for women with cervical dysplasia and other preinvasive genital tract conditions.

Most hysterectomies are undertaken for benign gynecologic diseases. Fewer operations are being undertaken for the following indications: leiomyoma, abnormal bleeding, benign ovarian mass, endometriosis, and pelvic organ prolapse. There has been great interest in alternative treatments that are conservative and usually nonsurgical. For example, uterine artery embolization is an alternative for the treatment of uterine fibroids. Pharmacologic therapies and ablative treatment are routinely offered as options for abnormal bleeding.

The many alternatives to performing an abdominal hysterectomy illustrate how well minimally invasive surgical techniques have been introduced. This issue highlights the different means for removing a uterus. Although vaginal hysterectomy has been performed for decades, laparoscopically assisted hysterectomy and total laparoscopic hysterectomy have been used since the 1990s. A robotic-assisted hysterectomy has become more widely accepted in the past decade.

Minimally invasive approaches to abdominal or vaginal hysterectomies offer many advantages and may be performed as outpatient procedures. As a result, the number

Obstet Gynecol Clin N Am 43 (2016) xi–xii
http://dx.doi.org/10.1016/j.ogc.2016.06.002
0889-8545/16/$ – see front matter © 2016 Published by Elsevier Inc.

obgyn.theclinics.com

of inpatient hysterectomies undertaken in the United States has declined to nearly half that performed nearly two decades ago. At the same time, there have been changes in referral patterns to surgeons performing many such general operations based on public reporting and quality initiatives. Efforts have focused on concentrating high-risk and specialized procedures to high-volume facilities and centers of excellence. For this reason, topics dealing with cesarean hysterectomy and uterine-preserving alternatives, enhanced recovery and improving outcomes, surgical simulation and competency, cost to the patient and hospital, and patient experience continue to gain in relevance.

I am grateful to the dedicated authors for their willingness to contribute to this very important issue. My special thanks go to Dr Occhino and Dr Trabuco, for their editorial assistance in selecting timely topics to be covered and in ensuring that the authors remain focused on what is evidence based. An update on this topic will be necessary for the reader in the next 10 years.

William F. Rayburn, MD, MBA
Continuing Medical Education
and Professional Development
Obstetrics and Gynecology
University of New Mexico School of Medicine
MSC 10 5580
1 University of New Mexico
Albuquerque, NM 87131-0001, USA

E-mail address:
Wrayburn@salud.unm.edu

Preface

Hysterectomy and the Alternatives

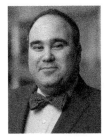 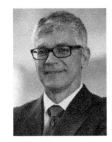

John A. Occhino, MD, MS   Emanuel C. Trabuco, MD, MS
Editors

We are excited to devote this entire issue of *Obstetrics and Gynecology Clinics of North America* to all aspects of hysterectomy. Despite recent trends showing decreasing numbers, hysterectomy remains one of the most common surgical procedures performed in North America. Nevertheless, since the mid-2000s, there has been a shift toward increasing robotic hysterectomy utilization. Although originally intended to replace abdominal hysterectomy, the introduction of robotic surgery has led to nationwide declines in all other approaches. This is despite the available evidence that vaginal hysterectomy is not only feasible in the vast majority of cases undergoing surgery for benign indications but also less expensive and less morbid when compared with other approaches, including robotic hysterectomy. These trends have been shown to have a negative impact on both resident training and postgraduate maintenance of surgical skills.

We begin with a discussion of alternatives to hysterectomy, specifically focusing on management of uterine fibroids and abnormal uterine bleeding. Next, individual routes of hysterectomy for benign disease are explored with a detailed description of techniques, applications, and complications for abdominal, vaginal, laparoscopic, and robotic approaches to hysterectomy written by experts in each category. We provide an evidence-focused review of the comparative literature among different modes of hysterectomy that not only dispel the myth of many commonly considered "contraindications" to vaginal surgery but also demonstrate that vaginal hysterectomy remains the safest and most cost-effective approach. Though rare, cesarean hysterectomy is often emergent and presents unique challenges to the obstetrician/gynecologist. We have chosen to dedicate an article to cesarean hysterectomy, presenting nonsurgical management of uterine atony in a stepwise manner. Subsequent criteria for reaching the decision point to move to peripartum hysterectomy are explored. Following hysterectomy discussions, we focus on evidence-based management of the fallopian tubes and ovaries at the time of benign hysterectomy, further exploring the role of

Obstet Gynecol Clin N Am 43 (2016) xiii–xiv
http://dx.doi.org/10.1016/j.ogc.2016.06.001
0889-8545/16/$ – see front matter © 2016 Published by Elsevier Inc.

salpingectomy in ovarian cancer prevention. Enhanced recovery, a novel and highly successful approach to the perioperative and postoperative management of the hysterectomy patient, is also presented, showing how changes introduced led to significant decreased length of stay, narcotic use, and hospital costs. As hysterectomy utilization continues to decline, surgical simulation will likely serve as an important adjunct to resident training and postgraduate maintenance of surgical skills. In this article, we describe the state-of-the-art in surgical simulation and provide tools for evaluation of surgical competency in various modes of hysterectomy. We finish with an article on current hot-topic issues facing the gynecologic surgeon, including uterine morcellation and reimbursement implications, with changing regulations following implementation of health care reform.

Our hope is that this issue provides readers with an evidence-based approach to the management of women with benign uterine disease: from uterine-preserving treatment to selecting the optimal management of adnexa and mode of uterine removal.

John A. Occhino, MD, MS
Department of Obstetrics and Gynecology
Division of Gynecologic Surgery
Mayo Clinic
200 First Street SW
Rochester, MN 55905, USA

Emanuel C. Trabuco, MD, MS
Department of Obstetrics and Gynecology
Division of Gynecologic Surgery
Mayo Clinic
200 First Street SW
Rochester, MN 55905, USA

E-mail addresses:
Occhino.john@mayo.edu (J.A. Occhino)
Trabuco.emanuel@mayo.edu (E.C. Trabuco)

Alternatives to Hysterectomy

Management of Uterine Fibroids

Shannon K. Laughlin-Tommaso, MD, MPH[a,b,*]

KEYWORDS

- Fibroids • Focused ultrasound ablation • Uterine artery embolization • Myomectomy
- Ulipristal acetate

KEY POINTS

- Fibroids are common and often asymptomatic.
- Treatment may be conservative and tailored to the symptoms.
- There are many alternatives to hysterectomy for fibroids including pharmacologic and nonpharmacologic approaches.
- Future directions in research may lead to preventative strategies that offer uterine and fertility preservation.

INTRODUCTION

Uterine fibroids are common, with up to 80% of women having radiologic or pathologic evidence of a fibroid by the time of menopause.[1,2] However, only 25% of women have symptoms severe enough to seek treatment. Fibroids may approximately impact health as well as social, physical, and work activities.[3] Studies have shown that the excess cost per woman with fibroids is over $4600, with loss of work costs averaging over $700 annually.[4]

Although hysterectomy is a definitive solution for symptomatic fibroids, many women would prefer to preserve their uterus for fertility and other reasons.[5] In fact, hysterectomy rates have decreased over the past decade with the increase in alternative treatments for fibroids and uterine bleeding.[6] However, there is little high-quality evidence comparing fibroid treatment options.[7]

Disclosure Statement: The author has received research funding, paid to Mayo Clinic, from Truven Health Analytics Inc and InSightec Ltd (Israel) for a focused ultrasonography ablation clinical trial. The author is on the data safety monitoring board for the Uterine Leiomyoma (fibroid) Treatment with Radiofrequency Ablation trial (ULTRA trial, Halt Medical, Inc).
[a] Department of Obstetrics and Gynecology, Mayo Clinic, 200 1st Street Southwest, Rochester, MN 55905, USA; [b] Department of Surgery, Mayo Clinic, 200 1st Street Southwest, Rochester, MN 55905, USA
* Department of Obstetrics and Gynecology, Mayo Clinic, 200 1st Street Southwest, Rochester, MN 55905.
E-mail address: Laughlintommaso.shannon@mayo.edu

Obstet Gynecol Clin N Am 43 (2016) 397–413
http://dx.doi.org/10.1016/j.ogc.2016.04.001
0889-8545/16/$ – see front matter
obgyn.theclinics.com

Because fibroids cause a range of symptoms (**Box 1**), a one-size fits all answer is not ideal. Care should be individualized to the patient to address her most pressing symptoms.[8] Women often have multiple tumors of varying size that can grow at different rates. Some have spontaneous regression; others grow steadily, and some increase quickly in short-lived growth spurts.[9,10] Thus, symptoms that are well-controlled for much of a woman's reproductive life may suddenly become more severe.

Fibroids also disproportionately affect African-American women. Tumors appear at a younger age in African American women than in Caucasian women.[11] In an ultrasound-screened population, prevalence of fibroids in women 18 to 30 years of age was 26% in black women and 7% in white women.[12] A national survey demonstrated that African American women were 2 to 3 times more likely to be concerned about fibroid treatments affecting fertility and pregnancy, likely because they encounter symptomatic fibroids while still child bearing.[3] Fibroids also tend to be larger and more numerous in African American women, which may limit options for alternative treatment.[11,12] For these reasons, uterine-preserving treatment options are necessary.

EVALUATION

Fibroids are identified often through clinical history and physical examination and then confirmed by ultrasound. However, asymptomatic fibroids may also be found incidentally on pelvic imaging. Deciding on a management strategy is based on whether the fibroids are causing symptoms. Fibroids that are asymptomatic do not require any treatment. Because fibroids will regress after menopause, expectant management is an option for some women.

If symptoms are present, the next step in management is to determine which symptoms are bothersome. Heavy menstrual bleeding (HMB) and painful periods are the most frequent symptoms and can be caused by fibroids that distort the uterine cavity (Type 0, 1, and 2 fibroids[13]) as well as larger intramural fibroids[14,15] (**Fig. 1**). A fibroid classification system was created to standardize the nomenclature of fibroids in practice and research.

The fibroid subclassification system can be described as follows[16]

- Type 0: completely intracavitary
- Type 1: less than 50% intramural (>=50% in the cavity)
- Type 2: at least 50% intramural (<50% in the cavity)
- Type 3: intramural but contacts endometrium

Box 1
Symptoms caused by uterine fibroids

Heavy menstrual bleeding

Pelvic pressure

Increased urinary frequency

Urinary retention

Bowel symptoms

Dyspareunia

Fertility issues (spontaneous abortion, decreased implantation)

Abdominal protrusion

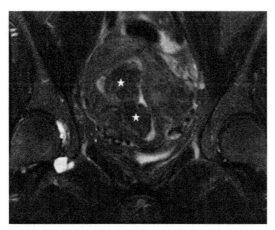

Fig. 1. Intracavitary submucosal (Type 0) fibroids labeled with stars in a woman with heavy menstrual bleeding as the only symptom (coronal view, MRI). Hysteroscopic resection provided symptom relief.

- Type 4: intramural
- Type 5: subserosal, but at least 50% intramural
- Type 6: subserosal, but less than 50% intramural
- Type 7: Subserosal Pedunculated
- Type 8: other (eg, cervical or parasitic)

Bulk symptoms most commonly include pelvic pressure, increased urinary frequency, urinary retention, constipation, and dyspareunia, which may occur with HMB or alone[17,18] (**Fig. 2**). Fibroid size is an important determinant of bulk symptoms; these unique tumors can grow to a large size at a rapid pace, but still remain benign.[10] Bulk symptoms usually occur from subserosal or pedunculated fibroids (Types 5, 6, and 7), but large intramural fibroids (Type 4) can also cause symptoms.

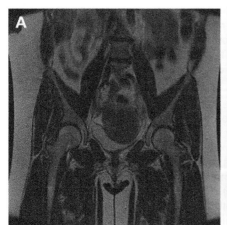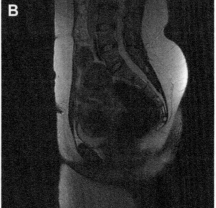

Fig. 2. T2-weighted images of (*A*) fibroid compressing the bladder (coronal view). (*B*) Anterior fibroid compressing bladder and posterior fibroid in contact with sacrum (sagittal view, large bowel distended possibly from proximal compression by fibroids).

Fertility may also be affected by fibroids. Fibroid location is the major determinant of the effect on fertility, followed by fibroid size. Evidence is strongest for fertility impairment for Types 0, 1, and 2 (submucosal) fibroids, but intramural fibroids that are greater than 5 cm may cause decreased implantation as well as higher frequency of spontaneous abortion.[19,20]

Pelvic examination can identify fibroids that distort the shape of the uterus (subserosal fibroids) or fibroids that are larger in size. Pelvic imaging helps to identify the size and number of fibroids. Ultrasound is a cost-effective and minimally invasive option for initial evaluation. Infusion of saline into the uterine cavity during ultrasound (sonohysterogram) helps to delineate the intracavitary extension of a submucosal fibroid to further plan surgery. Ultrasound is as sensitive as magnetic resonance imaging (MRI) for fibroids when there are fewer than 5 tumors, and uterine volume is under 375 mL.[21]

For larger uteri or numerous tumors, MRI can help delineate the size and location of fibroids. Contrast-enhanced MRI defines the blood flow to fibroids, which helps determine treatment options. MRI also outlines the proximity of fibroids to the uterine cavity, bladder, bowel, or sacrum, which may support the extent that symptoms can be attributed to the fibroids. Suspected submucosal fibroids may also be evaluated using hysteroscopy. Both office hysteroscopy and saline-infused ultrasound provide preoperative evaluation for hysteroscopic resection of fibroids.

MANAGEMENT GOALS

The management of uterine fibroids may include

- Reassurance
- Controlling symptoms
- Improving health and wellbeing
- Decreasing fibroid size or preventing further growth
- Transitioning into menopause without undergoing major surgery
- Optimizing fertility and pregnancy health

Asymptomatic Fibroids

Incidentally found fibroids that are not causing symptoms, especially after menopause, do not require treatment. Providing reassurance for these fibroids is an important aspect of care. There is no standard protocol for routine examinations or pelvic imaging for fibroids that are incidentally found. Repeat evaluation of the fibroids should be done if symptoms are identified or there are fertility concerns.

Heavy Menstrual Bleeding

HMB can be managed with either pharmacologic or nonpharmacologic options (**Box 2** and **Fig. 3**).

For women with fibroids that do not distort the uterine cavity, treatment of HMB includes medical therapy, hormonal implants, and endometrial ablation (See El-Nashar SA, Billow MR: Management of Abnormal Uterine Bleeding with Emphasis on Alternatives to Hysterectomy, in this issue). Nonhormonal medical therapies include nonsteroidal anti-inflammatory drugs (NSAIDs) and tranexamic acid, an oral antifibrinolytic. Both options require treatment only during the menstrual cycle and reduce bleeding up to 40%.[22] In a retrospective study, tranexamic acid was associated with necrosis in fibroids, but necrosis-related pain or decrease in fibroid size needs further research.[23]

> **Box 2**
> **Heavy menstrual bleeding management options**
>
> *Pharmacologic Strategies for HMB*
>
> Tranexamic Acid (antifibrinolytic)
>
> NSAIDs (mefanamic acid, naproxen)
>
> Combined estrogen–progestin contraceptives (eg, pills, ring, patch)
>
> Progestin only contraceptives (pills, shot, implant)
>
> Levonorgestrel intrauterine system
>
> *Nonpharmacologic Strategies for HMB*
>
> Hysteroscopic myomectomy
>
> Endometrial Ablation

Hormonal therapies include oral contraceptive pills, patches, rings, depot medroxyprogesterone acetate (DMPA), and levonorgestrel intrauterine systems (LNG-IUS, Mirena or Skyla, Bayer). Interestingly, while estrogen and progestins have been associated with fibroid development, oral contraceptive use is not associated with an increased risk of fibroids in most studies.[24,25] Early age at first use (younger than 17 years old) has been found to increase risk in 2 studies; however, early contraceptive use may indicate early exposure to sexually transmitted infections, which are hypothesized to increase fibroid incidence.[24–26] DMPA use reduces the risk of uterine fibroids in a dose-dependent fashion, from 20% lower risk in current users to 90% lower risk in women who used DMPA for more than 5 years.[27,28]

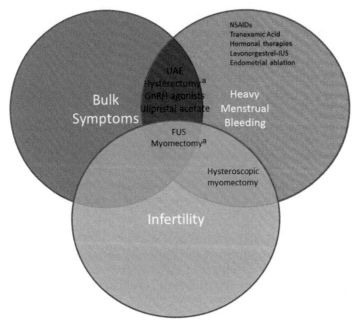

Fig. 3. Treatment options for fibroid symptoms. [a] Conventional laparoscopic, robotic-assisted laparoscopic, laparotomy (open).

One of the most effective medical therapies for control of HMB is the LNG-IUS; this intrauterine device reduces bleeding rates up to 80% and has high satisfaction among patients. Although highly effective for reduction in HMB, the LNG-IUS may have higher expulsion rates in women with fibroids (11%) than women without fibroids (3%).[29] Expulsion also increases with larger uterine cavities, a common effect of intramural fibroids. Saline-infused sonogram or hysteroscopy can ensure that fibroids are not distorting the uterine cavity prior to placement of LNG-IUS.

Endometrial ablation is a minimally invasive surgery that treats HMB by destroying the endometrium using various forms of energy: cryotherapy, microwave energy, radiofrequency energy, thermal balloon, or heated free fluid.[30] Some of these mechanisms, including microwave energy and thermal balloon, have been compared with resectoscopic ablation in randomized controlled trials, and worked best for uterine cavities with minimal distortion.[31,32] Fibroids were not associated with failure of endometrial ablation, but longer cavity lengths did increase failure rates.[33]

Hysteroscopic myomectomy

For women with submucosal fibroids (Types 0 and I), hysteroscopic myomectomy is a low-risk procedure with a quick recovery. Type 2 fibroids and fibroids greater than 3 cm increase the risk of incomplete resection and higher fluid absorption.[34,35] In these cases, a 2-stage procedure may be necessary. Hysteroscopic resection can be performed with electrosurgical resection using bipolar cautery or newer morcellator devices, which showed similar outcomes.[36] Perioperative complications include uterine perforation, fluid overload with subsequent hyponatremia, and intraoperative bleeding. Long-term risk of intrauterine adhesions after bipolar hysteroscopic resection was 7.5%.[37]

Hysteroscopic myomectomy has been shown to improve bleeding in 80% of women; bleeding is controlled in 95% of women if concomitant endometrial ablation is performed.[38] In 1 prospective study, risk of further surgery at 4 years was 21%, and satisfaction was greater than 70%.[35] The rate of fibroid recurrence is higher after larger or multiple fibroids compared with resection of solitary small fibroids.

Bulk Symptoms with or Without Heavy Menstrual Bleeding

For bulk symptoms with or without HMB, there are generally 2 options: shrinking or removing the fibroids (see **Fig. 3**).

Shrinking the fibroids can be done through pharmacologic treatments including GnRH agonists or antagonists and ulipristal acetate, a selective progesterone receptor modulator. Nonpharmacologic treatments that shrink fibroids to reduce bulk symptoms include magnetic resonance-guided focused ultrasound ablation (MRgFUS), uterine artery embolization (UAE), and laparoscopic radiofrequency volumetric thermal ablation (RFVTA). Removing the fibroids is done by myomectomy via a laparoscopic or open technique (**Box 3**).

GnRH agonists and antagonists

GnRH agonists and antagonists may be used preoperatively to improve anemia and decrease fibroid volume or may be used as a bridging therapy into menopause.[39] GnRH agonists initially increase the release of gonadotropins, which may causes a brief flare of HMB, then downregulate gonadotropins to a hypogonadal state similar to menopause. Leuprolide acetate has been US Food and Drug Administration (FDA)-approved for use in women with leiomyomas for preoperative treatment of anemia and fibroids. GnRH antagonists, which are currently marketed only for

---

Box 3
Treatment options for shrinking or removing fibroids

Pharmacologic Strategies

GnRH agonists/antagonists

Selective progesterone receptor modulators (Ulipristal acetate)[a]

Nonpharmacologic Strategies

Magnetic Resonance-guided Focused Ultrasound Ablation

Uterine Artery Embolization

Myomectomy

Radiofrequency volumetric thermal ablation

   [a] In Phase 3 trials in the United States currently; available in Canada and Europe.

---

ovulation induction, directly block gonadotropin effects, causing rapid clinical improvement without the initial flare. Data on long-term use with GnRH antagonists are limited.[40]

Benefits of GnRH analogues include amenorrhea and reduction in fibroid size during use. The decrease in HMB preoperatively improves blood counts and decreases anemia; this is valuable in the months prior to surgery to decrease the risk of blood transfusion.[39] Additionally, GnRH analogues have been shown to decrease the volume of the uterus up to 74%, improving the chances of a successful minimally invasive therapy, or in some cases, allowing for a laparoscopic approach instead of laparotomy.[41]

Unfortunately, GnRH analogues also have use-limiting adverse effects such as vasomotor symptoms and loss of bone mineral density. Add-back therapy in the form of progestin-only or estrogen–progestin combined therapy may ameliorate some of these adverse effects, but may limit the effects of the reduction in fibroid size.[42] Once GnRH analogues are discontinued, fibroids return to initial size, and symptoms return rapidly. Thus, long-term use of GnRH analogues is limited.

Ulipristal acetate

Several selective progesterone receptor modulators have been successful in reduction of fibroid size and symptoms, but have been limited by cystic glandular changes to the endometrium. Ulipristal acetate is currently available in Canada and Europe for treatment of uterine fibroids. Phase 3 clinical trials in the United States have shown that ulipristal acetate controls HMB in over 90% of women, decreases pain, and reduces fibroid size compared with placebo.[43]

Specifically, when ulipristal acetate was compared with placebo, several things were found:

- Over 40% of women had 25% or greater reduction in fibroid size
- 30% of women had 25% or greater reduction in uterine size
- Over 70% of women achieved amenorrhea
- There was an increase in hemoglobin levels greater for ulipristal acetate than placebo

The adverse effect profile of ulipristal acetate is similar to that of the placebo group, with only a few serious adverse events, mainly uterine or ovarian hemorrhage, in the treatment arm.[43] Unlike GnRH agonist therapy, estradiol levels remained in the follicular phase range during treatment with ulipristal acetate. Although nonphysiologic changes did occur in the endometrium, no premalignant or malignant changes were seen. These changes were reversible after treatment completion even in women who underwent 4 consecutive 12-week courses of ulipristal acetate therapy.[44]

When compared with leuprolide acetate, ulipristal acetate had equivalent control of bleeding, but time to amenorrhea was quicker for ulipristal acetate and vasomotor symptoms significantly less.[45] Leuprolide acetate caused significantly greater uterine volume reduction and higher, but similar, fibroid volume reduction. However, fibroid volume reduction was more sustained for ulipristal acetate, which is promising as an option for intermittent medical treatment of fibroids. Two randomized controlled trials have tested the effects of repeated 3-month courses of ulipristal acetate and found that subsequent treatment periods have improved bleeding control and reduction in fibroid volume.[44,46] This provides the first option for a long-term preventative pharmacologic management for uterine fibroids.

Nonpharmacologic Strategies

Magnetic resonance-guided focused ultrasound ablation

Magnetic resonance-guided focused ultrasound ablation (MRgFUS) is a minimally invasive therapy that uses ultrasound energy directed through the abdominal wall (no incisions required) under real-time MRI monitoring to shrink fibroids (**Fig. 4**).[47] The energy causes coagulative necrosis of the fibroids, which then lose perfusion and shrink in size, decreasing symptoms. The fibroids are not completely removed and will remain present; the reduction in size of the fibroids is not correlated to the symptom relief, which tends to be high.

MRgFUS continues to grow in popularity because of high patient satisfaction, minimal adverse effects, and speedy recovery.[48] Treatment lasts approximately 3 hours per day with some uteri requiring 2 consecutive days of treatments. Fibroids up to 10 cm in diameter or several medium-sized fibroids are routinely treated. Women return to work within days of treatment and usually do not require narcotic pain medication. Treatment may be limited by extensive abdominal wall scarring or bowel lying between the abdominal wall and the uterus. Major contraindications are metal implants, defibrillators, or other contraindications to undergoing MRI.

Optimal results are achieved when the majority of the fibroid can be treated, as determined by the nonperfused volume (NPV) ratio at the end of treatment.[49] Even with less than 20% of the fibroid volume treated, symptom severity scores significantly

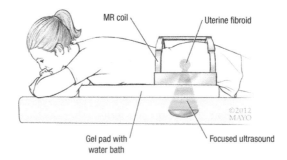

MR coil   Uterine fibroid

©2012 MAYO

Gel pad with water bath   Focused ultrasound

The ultrasound equipment is below the table.
It directs sound waves up into your abdomen.

Fig. 4. Focused ultrasound ablation procedure for treatment of uterine fibroids. (*Used with permission of Mayo Foundation for Medical Education and Research, Rochester, MN. All rights reserved.*)

dropped and remained low for 24 months. Higher NPV has also been shown to be predictive of better outcomes and no increase in adverse events.[50] More experience with MRgFUS and advances in devices will continue to improve NPV. Newer devices have demonstrated NPVs of 88% (38%–100%).[51] Fibroid consistency also determines NPV and outcomes. Fibroids with higher vascularity and more cellular tissue tend to have lower NPV and higher reintervention rates.[50,52]

Reintervention for fibroids is used to determine success of the minimally invasive treatments; for MRgFUS, reintervention occurs in about 23% of women after 4 years.[52] Because MRgFUS treats individual fibroids, there may be other small fibroids that cannot be successfully treated or locations that are inaccessible. Reperfusion of treated fibroids may also occur with time. Clinical predictors of success include older age, more fibroids, and higher fibroid volume.[53]

Uterine artery embolization (or uterine fibroid embolization)

UAE is a nonsurgical therapy that shrinks fibroids via blocking arterial blood flow to the fibroids. UAE is performed under conscious sedation; femoral vessels are accessed through a small incision in the groin. Using fluoroscopic guidance, a catheter is passed through the uterine arteries, and embolic agents are targeted at the symptomatic fibroids (**Fig. 5**). The goal is to decrease blood flow, causing infarction and eventual

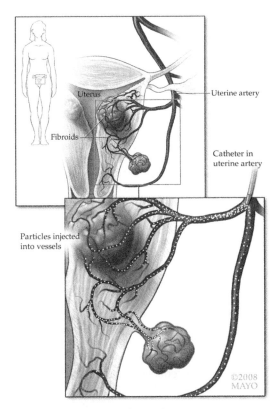

Uterine artery embolization

Fig. 5. Uterine artery embolization procedure for treatment of uterine fibroids. (*Used with permission of Mayo Foundation for Medical Education and Research, Rochester, MN. All rights reserved.*)

shrinking of the fibroids. Similar to MRgFUS, symptom control may be high even with small reduction in fibroid size. Women have a significantly faster return to work than with surgical treatment of fibroids.[54]

Most fibroid uteri are good candidates for UAE. Solitary fibroids more than 10 cm or multiple fibroids with a uterine volume consistent with a 20-week or greater gestation are considered relative contraindications to UAE, but successful treatment can be accomplished.[55] Prior surgeries and adhesions are not problematic for UAE, but vascular disease may limit access to the vessels. Ovarian impairment may occur after UAE, especially in older women, and may be an asset for perimenopausal women seeking relief from HMB.[56]

UAE has been shown to have equivalent reduction in symptoms, improvement in quality of life, and lower risk of infection than hysterectomy.[54] Two randomized clinical trials in Europe have shown long-lasting symptom control for up to 5 years with improvement in bleeding, pain, and bulk symptoms.[54,57]

Reintervention for UAE is similar to MRgFUS outcomes. Reintervention rates have been documented as 9% at 1 year and 28% at 5 years from randomized controlled trials of UAE versus surgery.[54,57] The first randomized controlled trial comparing UAE and MRgFUS has completed enrollment, and long-term results are being analyzed (FIRSTT trial, clinicaltrials.gov # NCT00995878).[58]

Laparoscopic radiofrequency volumetric thermal ablation

RFVTA is a safe and effective treatment FDA-approved in 2012 for women who desire uterine conservation and quick recovery.[59] The procedure is performed under laparoscopic guidance using a laparoscopic ultrasound probe to delineate fibroids and a percutaneous radiofrequency handpiece with a deployable electrode array. Fibroid mapping is performed using the laparoscopic ultrasound, and real-time imaging monitors insertion of the electrodes into the fibroids. The fibroids are ablated and the insertion tract coagulated on removal.

Outcomes from clinical trials are still short-term for RFVTA, but they show promising results for controlling symptoms and improving quality of life out to 2 years.[59] In a randomized trial comparing RFVTA with laparoscopic myomectomy, treatment time was similar, but women who underwent RFVTA had a higher percentage of fibroids treated (98.6% vs 80.3%), less intraoperative blood loss, and shorter hospital stays.[60]

Abdominal myomectomy

Myomectomy, or removal of fibroids, is still considered the gold standard for women who want to preserve their fertility, but the procedure has known risks for pregnancy, including adhesion formation, anemia, risk of hysterectomy, and increased risk of uterine rupture.[61] Myomectomy can be performed laparoscopically with or without robotic assistance or using an open abdominal technique.

Location and size of fibroids are important in determining the best route for surgical removal. Laparoscopic myomectomy, which works best for subserosal and large intramural fibroids, reduces recovery time, decreases postoperative pain, and decreases postoperative fever compared with open procedures.[62] Robotic assistance is associated with fewer intraoperative complications and less blood loss, but longer operative times.[63]

Laparotomy is advantageous in reducing residual fibroid burden when removing multiple small intramural fibroids. In addition, laparotomy is often better in uteri that rise above the umbilicus, making laparoscopic approach more difficult.[63]

Special consideration: morcellation

A new issue that limits laparoscopic and robotic myomectomy is a new FDA black box warning on laparoscopic power morcellators. Intraperitoneal morcellation, whether hand or power morcellation, has been shown in retrospective studies to increase the risk of local recurrence of unsuspected leiomyosarcoma, which decreases survival.[64,65] Some argue that power morcellation should not be singled out; any disruption of an unsuspected leiomyosarcoma, including myomectomy or supracervical hysterectomy, could upstage the disease.[66,67] However, many counter this argument that eliminating these lower-risk options is not ethical given the low incidence of leiomyosarcoma.[67]

The true risk of unsuspected leiomyosarcoma among presumed fibroids remains controversial and is age-related. Many gynecologic specialists are advocating for continued, but conservative use of the morcellator preserving the laparoscopic approach, especially in young women.[67] When compared with laparotomy, the laparoscopic route reduces both surgical risks and overall mortality.[68]

REPRODUCTION AND FIBROIDS

Fibroids are associated with infertility and pregnancy complications, but treatment of fibroids to improve fertility can be complicated. Having a fibroid is the only abnormal finding in less than 3% of women with infertility.[69] Thus, other causes of infertility should be evaluated. In addition, approximately 5% of women with infertility will have a fibroid, and in a study that screened women with ultrasound in the first trimester, 11% of pregnant women had fibroids.[11]

Most studies agree that submucosal fibroids are associated with infertility and spontaneous abortion. Types 0, 1, and 2 fibroids have the highest fertility risks, with approximately a 70% decrease in clinical pregnancy rate, implantation rate, and live birth rate.[70] Spontaneous abortion was increased about 70% in women with submucosal fibroids. For submucosal fibroids, hysteroscopic myomectomy often improves outcomes with few fertility-inhibiting adverse effects.

There is more controversy as to the effect of intramural fibroids. In the systematic review by Pritts and colleagues,[70] intramural fibroids reduced pregnancy rates and increased spontaneous abortion rates, but to a lesser extent than submucosal fibroids. However, most of the included studies had inadequate evaluation of the cavity to rule out a submucosal component. In studies that used hysteroscopy, only implantation rate remained significantly decreased.[70] Removal of intramural fibroids for fertility did not significantly improve pregnancy rates.[71] Risks of myomectomy, such as postoperative adhesions, uterine rupture, and the rare case of hysterectomy, may outweigh the benefits of removing an intramural fibroid.

For fibroids affecting fertility, risks and benefits of all fibroid treatment options should be discussed and patient autonomy respected, especially for women with increased surgical risks. UAE and MRgFUS may be alternatives to myomectomy for some patients. In addition to the age-related risk of ovarian impairment, UAE is associated with placental abnormalities.[72,73] In a large cohort study, there was approximately a 12% risk of placental abnormalities after UAE; 2 of the 3 cases were at risk due to advanced maternal age, but none had prior myomectomy or cesarean section.[72] Nonetheless, many women have had healthy pregnancies after uterine artery embolization.

Reports of reproductive outcomes after MRgFUS are encouraging. In 1 study of pregnancy after MRgFUS, 54 pregnancies in 51 women were reported.[74]

Live birth occurred in 41% of pregnancies (with an additional 21% ongoing beyond 30 weeks); vaginal delivery rate was 64%, and there were no low-birth-weight infants. Complications were similar to the general pregnant population, including 2 placental abnormalities in women with known risk factors. As a result, the FDA-approved indication for MRgFUS has been updated to include women who desire future fertility after appropriate counseling. Limited reproductive outcomes following RFVTA also indicate success, with 5 of 6 women delivering full-term healthy infants and 1 having a spontaneous miscarriage.[75]

Pregnancy complications have been attributed to fibroids in many retrospective studies. In a population-based study in Taiwan, women with fibroids had a 4% higher risk of preterm birth and a 1.7% higher risk of small for gestational age infants (14.7 g lower birthweight).[76] Similarly, Shavell and colleagues[77] found that women with fibroids greater than 5 cm delivered approximately 2 weeks earlier than women without fibroids or women with fibroids no bigger than 5 cm. Short cervix, preterm premature rupture of membranes, cesarean section, and malpresentation are some of the other complications attributed to fibroids. The advantage of these 2 studies is that the controls also had an ultrasound to confirm there were no fibroids. Retrospective study results for fibroids may be confounded by ascertainment bias.[69]

Interestingly, pregnancy helps to reduce the risk of fibroids. Uterine remodeling following pregnancy seems to preferentially shrink or eliminate fibroids. In an ultrasound-based study of 171 pregnant women with at least 1 fibroid, 36% of fibroids were not visible on postpartum ultrasound and 80% of the remaining fibroids decreased in size.[78] Age at first pregnancy, and time since last pregnancy also influences risk of fibroids (**Table 1**).[24,79]

Table 1 Self-management strategies		
Strategy	**Type/Amount**	**Effect**
Physical activity	≥7 h/wk v <2 h/wk	40% reduction in fibroid risk
Diet	1. Plant-based 2. High red meat/ham 3. High soy diet 4. Dairy (≥4 v <1 serving/d)	1. Reduces fibroid risk 2. Increases fibroid risk 3. No difference 4. 30% lower risk
Body mass index/weight gain	1. Overweight and obesity 2. Weight gain of ≥10 kg	1. Increases with overweight, but not obesity in some studies 2. 16%–23% increased risk
Parity	1. Parous v nulliparous 2. Time since last birth	1. 2%–50% reduction in risk 2. Higher risk with longer time since last birth
Stress	Racism or early life abuse	Higher incidence of fibroids
Environmental contaminants (endocrine disruptors)	1. Dioxin 2. Polychlorinated biphenyls 3. Bisphenol A	1. Reduced risk of fibroids 2 & 3. Increased risk in some studies
Vitamin D supplementation	—	20% reduction in fibroid risk for each 10 ng/mL increase in vitamin D levels

From Wise LA, Laughlin-Tommaso SK. Epidemiology of uterine fibroids: from menarche to menopause. Clin Obstet Gynecol 2016;59(1):2–24; with permission.

SUMMARY/DISCUSSION

Fibroids are common and can occur in some women at a young age, threatening future fertility. Treatment can be tailored to treat a range of symptoms while maintaining the patient's desire to preserve fertility. Several minimally invasive techniques allow for a quick recovery, and medical therapy is on the horizon that both treats symptoms and may be used for prevention. Reassurance that fibroids will become asymptomatic after menopause provides a woman the freedom to choose expectant management or lesser invasive options that will bridge her until menopause. Hysterectomy, while definitive, is not required.

REFERENCES

1. Day Baird D, Dunson DB, Hill MC, et al. High cumulative incidence of uterine leiomyoma in black and white women: ultrasound evidence. Am J Obstet Gynecol 2003;188(1):100–7.
2. Cramer SF, Patel A. The frequency of uterine leiomyomas. Am J Clin Pathol 1990; 94(4):435–8.
3. Stewart EA, Nicholson WK, Bradley L, et al. The burden of uterine fibroids for African-American women: results of a national survey. J Womens Health (Larchmt) 2013;22(10):807–16.
4. Hartmann KE, Birnbaum H, Ben-Hamadi R, et al. Annual costs associated with diagnosis of uterine leiomyomata. Obstet Gynecol 2006;108(4):930–7.
5. Borah BJ, Nicholson WK, Bradley L, et al. The impact of uterine leiomyomas: a national survey of affected women. Am J Obstet Gynecol 2013;209(4):319.e1–20.
6. Wright JD, Herzog TJ, Tsui J, et al. Nationwide trends in the performance of inpatient hysterectomy in the United States. Obstet Gynecol 2013;122(2 Pt 1):233–41.
7. Viswanathan M, Hartmann K, McKoy N, et al. Management of uterine fibroids: an update of the evidence. Evid Rep Technol Assess (Full Rep) 2007;(154):1–122.
8. Laughlin SK, Stewart EA. Uterine leiomyomas: individualizing the approach to a heterogeneous condition. Obstet Gynecol 2011;117(2 Pt 1):396–403.
9. Peddada SD, Laughlin SK, Miner K, et al. Growth of uterine leiomyomata among premenopausal black and white women. Proc Natl Acad Sci U S A 2008;105(50): 19887–92.
10. Baird DD, Garrett TA, Laughlin SK, et al. Short-term change in growth of uterine leiomyoma: tumor growth spurts. Fertil Steril 2011;95(1):242–6.
11. Laughlin SK, Baird DD, Savitz DA, et al. Prevalence of uterine leiomyomas in the first trimester of pregnancy: an ultrasound-screening study. Obstet Gynecol 2009;113(3):630–5.
12. Marsh EE, Ekpo GE, Cardozo ER, et al. Racial differences in fibroid prevalence and ultrasound findings in asymptomatic young women (18-30 years old): a pilot study. Fertil Steril 2013;99(7):1951–7.
13. Wamsteker K, Emanuel MH, de Kruif JH. Transcervical hysteroscopic resection of submucous fibroids for abnormal uterine bleeding: results regarding the degree of intramural extension. Obstet Gynecol 1993;82(5):736–40.
14. Puri K, Famuyide AO, Erwin PJ, et al. Submucosal fibroids and the relation to heavy menstrual bleeding and anemia. Am J Obstet Gynecol 2014;210(1):38.e1–7.
15. Wegienka G, Baird DD, Hertz-Picciotto I, et al. Self-reported heavy bleeding associated with uterine leiomyomata. Obstet Gynecol 2003;101(3):431–7.
16. Munro MG, Critchley HO, Broder MS, et al. FIGO classification system (PALM-COEIN) for causes of abnormal uterine bleeding in nongravid women of reproductive age. Int J Gynaecol Obstet 2011;113(1):3–13.

17. Wu CQ, Lefebvre G, Frecker H, et al. Urinary retention and uterine leiomyomas: a case series and systematic review of the literature. Int Urogynecol J 2015;26(9): 1277–84.

18. Laughlin-Tommaso SK, Borah BJ, Stewart EA. Effect of menses on standardized assessment of sexual dysfunction among women with uterine fibroids: a cohort study. Fertil Steril 2015;104(2):435–9.

19. Oliveira FG, Abdelmassih VG, Diamond MP, et al. Impact of subserosal and intramural uterine fibroids that do not distort the endometrial cavity on the outcome of in vitro fertilization-intracytoplasmic sperm injection. Fertil Steril 2004;81(3):582–7.

20. American College of Obstetricians and Gynecologists. ACOG practice bulletin. Alternatives to hysterectomy in the management of leiomyomas. Obstet Gynecol 2008;112(2 Pt 1):387–400.

21. Dueholm M, Lundorf E, Hansen ES, et al. Accuracy of magnetic resonance imaging and transvaginal ultrasonography in the diagnosis, mapping, and measurement of uterine myomas. Am J Obstet Gynecol 2002;186(3):409–15.

22. Lukes AS, Moore KA, Muse KN, et al. Tranexamic acid treatment for heavy menstrual bleeding: a randomized controlled trial. Obstet Gynecol 2010;116(4):865–75.

23. Ip PP, Lam KW, Cheung CL, et al. Tranexamic acid-associated necrosis and intralesional thrombosis of uterine leiomyomas: a clinicopathologic study of 147 cases emphasizing the importance of drug-induced necrosis and early infarcts in leiomyomas. Am J Surg Pathol 2007;31(8):1215–24.

24. Wise LA, Palmer JR, Harlow BL, et al. Reproductive factors, hormonal contraception, and risk of uterine leiomyomata in African-American women: a prospective study. Am J Epidemiol 2004;159(2):113–23.

25. Marshall LM, Spiegelman D, Goldman MB, et al. A prospective study of reproductive factors and oral contraceptive use in relation to the risk of uterine leiomyomata. Fertil Steril 1998;70(3):432–9.

26. Laughlin SK, Schroeder JC, Baird DD. New directions in the epidemiology of uterine fibroids. Semin Reprod Med 2010;28(3):204–17.

27. Harmon QE, Baird DD. Use of depot medroxyprogesterone acetate and prevalent leiomyoma in young African American women. Hum Reprod 2015;30(6): 1499–504.

28. Lumbiganon P, Rugpao S, Phandhu-fung S, et al. Protective effect of depot-medroxyprogesterone acetate on surgically treated uterine leiomyomas: a multicentre case–control study. Br J Obstet Gynaecol 1996;103(9):909–14.

29. Zapata LB, Whiteman MK, Tepper NK, et al. Intrauterine device use among women with uterine fibroids: a systematic review. Contraception 2010;82(1):41–55.

30. ACOG Committee on Practice Bulletins. ACOG Practice Bulletin. Clinical management guidelines for obstetrician-gynecologists. Number 81, May 2007. Obstet Gynecol 2007;109(5):1233–48.

31. Cooper KG, Bain C, Parkin DE. Comparison of microwave endometrial ablation and transcervical resection of the endometrium for treatment of heavy menstrual loss: a randomized trial. Lancet 1999;354(9193):1859–63.

32. Soysal ME, Soysal SK, Vicdan K. Thermal balloon ablation in myoma-induced menorrhagia under local anesthesia. Gynecol Obstet Invest 2001;51(2):128–33.

33. El-Nashar SA, Hopkins MR, Creedon DJ, et al. Prediction of treatment outcomes after global endometrial ablation. Obstet Gynecol 2009;113(1):97–106.

34. Emanuel MH, Hart A, Wamsteker K, et al. An analysis of fluid loss during transcervical resection of submucous myomas. Fertil Steril 1997;68(5):881–6.

35. Hart R, Molnar BG, Magos A. Long term follow up of hysteroscopic myomectomy assessed by survival analysis. Br J Obstet Gynaecol 1999;106(7):700–5.

36. Hamidouche A, Vincienne M, Thubert T, et al. Operative hysteroscopy for myoma removal: morcellation versus bipolar loop resection. J Gynecol Obstet Biol Reprod (Paris) 2015;44(7):658–64 [in French].

37. Touboul C, Fernandez H, Deffieux X, et al. Uterine synechiae after bipolar hysteroscopic resection of submucosal myomas in patients with infertility. Fertil Steril 2009;92(5):1690–3.

38. Loffer FD. Improving results of hysteroscopic submucosal myomectomy for menorrhagia by concomitant endometrial ablation. J Minim Invasive Gynecol 2005;12(3):254–60.

39. Lethaby A, Vollenhoven B, Sowter M. Efficacy of pre-operative gonadotrophin hormone releasing analogues for women with uterine fibroids undergoing hysterectomy or myomectomy: a systematic review. BJOG 2002;109(10):1097–108.

40. Minaguchi H, Wong JM, Snabes MC. Clinical use of nafarelin in the treatment of leiomyomas. A review of the literature. J Reprod Med 2000;45(6):481–9.

41. Carr BR, Marshburn PB, Weatherall PT, et al. An evaluation of the effect of gonadotropin-releasing hormone analogs and medroxyprogesterone acetate on uterine leiomyomata volume by magnetic resonance imaging: a prospective, randomized, double blind, placebo-controlled, crossover trial. J Clin Endocrinol Metab 1993;76(5):1217–23.

42. Mizutani T, Sugihara A, Honma H, et al. Effect of steroid add-back therapy on the proliferative activity of uterine leiomyoma cells under gonadotropin-releasing hormone agonist therapy. Gynecol Endocrinol 2005;20(2):80–3.

43. Donnez J, Tatarchuk TF, Bouchard P, et al. Ulipristal acetate versus placebo for fibroid treatment before surgery. N Engl J Med 2012;366(5):409–20.

44. Donnez J, Donnez O, Matule D, et al. Long-term medical management of uterine fibroids with ulipristal acetate. Fertil Steril 2016;105(1):165–73.

45. Donnez J, Tomaszewski J, Vazquez F, et al. Ulipristal acetate versus leuprolide acetate for uterine fibroids. N Engl J Med 2012;366(5):421–32.

46. Donnez J, Arriagada P, Donnez O, et al. Current management of myomas: the place of medical therapy with the advent of selective progesterone receptor modulators. Curr Opin Obstet Gynecol 2015;27(6):422–31.

47. Hesley GK, Gorny KR, Henrichsen TL, et al. A clinical review of focused ultrasound ablation with magnetic resonance guidance: an option for treating uterine fibroids. Ultrasound Q 2008;24(2):131–9.

48. Stewart EA, Gostout B, Rabinovici J, et al. Sustained relief of leiomyoma symptoms by using focused ultrasound surgery. Obstet Gynecol 2007;110(2 Pt 1): 279–87.

49. Yoon SW, Lee C, Cha SH, et al. Patient selection guidelines in MR-guided focused ultrasound surgery of uterine fibroids: a pictorial guide to relevant findings in screening pelvic MRI. Eur Radiol 2008;18(12):2997–3006.

50. Quinn SD, Vedelago J, Gedroyc W, et al. Safety and five-year re-intervention following magnetic resonance-guided focused ultrasound (MRgFUS) for uterine fibroids. Eur J Obstet Gynecol Reprod Biol 2014;182:247–51.

51. Trumm CG, Stahl R, Clevert DA, et al. Magnetic resonance imaging-guided focused ultrasound treatment of symptomatic uterine fibroids: impact of technology advancement on ablation volumes in 115 patients. Invest Radiol 2013;48(6): 359–65.

52. Gorny KR, Borah BJ, Brown DL, et al. Incidence of additional treatments in women treated with MR-guided focused US for symptomatic uterine fibroids: review of 138 patients with an average follow-up of 2.8 years. J Vasc Interv Radiol 2014;25(10):1506–12.

53. Gorny KR, Borah BJ, Weaver AL, et al. Clinical predictors of successful magnetic resonance-guided focused ultrasound (MRgFUS) for uterine leiomyoma. J Ther Ultrasound 2013;1:15.

54. van der Kooij SM, Hehenkamp WJ, Volkers NA, et al. Uterine artery embolization vs hysterectomy in the treatment of symptomatic uterine fibroids: 5-year outcome from the randomized EMMY trial. Am J Obstet Gynecol 2010;203(2):105.e1–13.

55. Smeets AJ, Nijenhuis RJ, van Rooij WJ, et al. Uterine artery embolization in patients with a large fibroid burden: long-term clinical and MR follow-up. Cardiovasc Intervent Radiol 2010;33(5):943–8.

56. Katsumori T, Kasahara T, Tsuchida Y, et al. Amenorrhea and resumption of menstruation after uterine artery embolization for fibroids. Int J Gynaecol Obstet 2008;103(3):217–21.

57. Edwards RD, Moss JG, Lumsden MA, et al. Uterine-artery embolization versus surgery for symptomatic uterine fibroids. N Engl J Med 2007;356(4):360–70.

58. Bouwsma EV, Hesley GK, Woodrum DA, et al. Comparing focused ultrasound and uterine artery embolization for uterine fibroids-rationale and design of the Fibroid Interventions: reducing symptoms today and tomorrow (FIRSTT) trial. Fertil Steril 2011;96(3):704–10.

59. Guido RS, Macer JA, Abbott K, et al. Radiofrequency volumetric thermal ablation of fibroids: a prospective, clinical analysis of two years' outcome from the Halt trial. Health Qual Life Outcomes 2013;11:139.

60. Brucker SY, Hahn M, Kraemer D, et al. Laparoscopic radiofrequency volumetric thermal ablation of fibroids versus laparoscopic myomectomy. Int J Gynaecol Obstet 2014;125(3):261–5.

61. Stewart EA. Clinical practice. Uterine fibroids. N Engl J Med 2015;372(17):1646–55.

62. Bhave Chittawar P, Franik S, Pouwer AW, et al. Minimally invasive surgical techniques versus open myomectomy for uterine fibroids. Cochrane Database Syst Rev 2014;(10):CD004638.

63. Griffin L, Feinglass J, Garrett A, et al. Postoperative outcomes after robotic versus abdominal myomectomy. Jsls 2013;17(3):407–13.

64. George S, Barysauskas C, Serrano C, et al. Retrospective cohort study evaluating the impact of intraperitoneal morcellation on outcomes of localized uterine leiomyosarcoma. Cancer 2014;120(20):3154–8.

65. Oduyebo T, Rauh-Hain AJ, Meserve EE, et al. The value of re-exploration in patients with inadvertently morcellated uterine sarcoma. Gynecol Oncol 2014;132(2):360–5.

66. Pritts EA, Parker WH, Brown J, et al. Outcome of occult uterine leiomyosarcoma after surgery for presumed uterine fibroids: a systematic review. J Minim Invasive Gynecol 2015;22(1):26–33.

67. Parker WH, Kaunitz AM, Pritts EA, et al. U.S. Food and Drug administration's guidance regarding morcellation of leiomyomas: well-intentioned, but is it harmful for women? Obstet Gynecol 2016;127(1):18–22.

68. Siedhoff MT, Wheeler SB, Rutstein SE, et al. Laparoscopic hysterectomy with morcellation vs abdominal hysterectomy for presumed fibroid tumors in premenopausal women: a decision analysis. Am J Obstet Gynecol 2015;212(5):591.e1–8.

69. Olive DL, Pritts EA. Fibroids and reproduction. Semin Reprod Med 2010;28(3):218–27.

70. Pritts EA, Parker WH, Olive DL. Fibroids and infertility: an updated systematic review of the evidence. Fertil Steril 2009;91(4):1215–23.

71. Casini ML, Rossi F, Agostini R, et al. Effects of the position of fibroids on fertility. Gynecol Endocrinol 2006;22(2):106–9.
72. Pron G, Mocarski E, Bennett J, et al. Pregnancy after uterine artery embolization for leiomyomata: the Ontario multicenter trial. Obstet Gynecol 2005;105(1):67–76.
73. Hehenkamp WJ, Volkers NA, Broekmans FJ, et al. Loss of ovarian reserve after uterine artery embolization: a randomized comparison with hysterectomy. Hum Reprod 2007;22(7):1996–2005.
74. Rabinovici J, David M, Fukunishi H, et al. Pregnancy outcome after magnetic resonance-guided focused ultrasound surgery (MRgFUS) for conservative treatment of uterine fibroids. Fertil Steril 2010;93(1):199–209.
75. Berman JM, Bolnick JM, Pemueller RR, et al. Reproductive Outcomes in women following radiofrequency volumetric thermal ablation of symptomatic fibroids. A retrospective case series analysis. J Reprod Med 2015;60(5–6):194–8.
76. Chen YH, Lin HC, Chen SF. Increased risk of preterm births among women with uterine leiomyoma: a nationwide population-based study. Hum Reprod 2009;24(12):3049–56.
77. Shavell VI, Thakur M, Sawant A, et al. Adverse obstetric outcomes associated with sonographically identified large uterine fibroids. Fertil Steril 2012;97(1):107–10.
78. Laughlin SK, Herring AH, Savitz DA, et al. Pregnancy-related fibroid reduction. Fertil Steril 2010;94(6):2421–3.
79. Baird DD, Dunson DB. Why is parity protective for uterine fibroids? Epidemiology 2003;14(2):247–50.

Management of Abnormal Uterine Bleeding with Emphasis on Alternatives to Hysterectomy

Megan R. Billow, DO[a,b], Sherif A. El-Nashar, MD, PhD[a,b,c],*

KEYWORDS

- Abnormal uterine bleeding • Heavy menstrual bleeding • Endometrial ablation • IUD
- Medical management

KEY POINTS

- Abnormal uterine bleeding (AUB) negatively impacts a woman's quality of life. After exclusion of pregnancy, the initial evaluation includes a complete history and physical examination focusing on endometrial cancer risks, screening for an underlying coagulopathy, and review of medications that may contribute to AUB.
- Following the initial evaluation, medical management includes oral hormonal or nonhormonal treatments.
- If AUB persists, a more comprehensive evaluation of the uterine cavity for structural abnormalities based on the PALM-COEIN system is necessary to guide management. The levonorgestrel intrauterine system is a safe and effective therapy for women with AUB who desire contraception. With proper patient selection, an endometrial ablation (EA) is a minimally invasive surgical option with low risk and can significantly decrease heavy menstrual bleeding, improve quality of life, and avoid a hysterectomy.

INTRODUCTION

Abnormal uterine bleeding (AUB) is a common complaint of women. It affects 10% to 15% of reproductive-aged women, accounts for up to 30% of outpatient office visits annually, and costs the US health care system more than $2 billion annually.[1] It is defined as any deviation from a normal menstrual cycle including changes in the frequency, duration, and amount of bleeding. AUB negatively impacts a woman's

[a] Department of Obstetrics and Gynecology and Reproductive Biology, University Hospitals, Case Medical Center, Cleveland, OH, USA; [b] Department of Reproductive Biology, University Hospitals, Case Medical Center, Cleveland, OH, USA; [c] Department of Obstetrics and Gynecology, Assiut University, Assiut, Egypt
* Corresponding author. Division of Female Pelvic Medicine and Reconstructive Surgery, Department of Obstetrics and Gynecology, University Hospitals, Case Medical Center, Mailstop: MAC 5034, 11100 Euclid Avenue, Cleveland, OH 44106-5047.
E-mail address: sherif.el-nashar@uhhospitals.org

Obstet Gynecol Clin N Am 43 (2016) 415–430
http://dx.doi.org/10.1016/j.ogc.2016.04.002
0889-8545/16/$ – see front matter © 2016 Elsevier Inc. All rights reserved.

health-related quality of life including sexual, emotional, financial, and professional life.[1,2] In 2011, an expert group from the International Federation of Gynecology and Obstetrics Working Group on Menstrual Disorders proposed the PALM-COEIN classification of AUB (polyp, adenomyosis, leiomyoma, and malignancy and hyperplasia; coagulopathy, ovulatory dysfunction, endometrial, iatrogenic, and not yet classified). This platform facilitates communication related to the cause, evaluation, and management of AUB for clinical and research purposes.[3]

The initial treatment is generally medical management in the form of systemic hormonal and nonhormonal medications. These only result in a 40% to 50% reduction of menstrual blood loss (MBL). Furthermore, both treatments are associated with a high rate of noncompliance. Irrespective of the underlying cause, a hysterectomy is the definitive treatment of AUB. However, it is associated with significant risks, such as bleeding; infection; thromboembolic events; and injury to intestines, bladder, and ureters.[4–9] A hysterectomy is also associated with higher costs, longer operating time, and higher risks for postoperative morbidity. Uterine-preserving options, such as the levonorgestrel intrauterine system (LNG-IUS) and endometrial ablation (EA), provide less invasive alternatives to hysterectomy.[10,11]

This article discusses the initial evaluation and management of AUB. Also discussed are the follow-up and further management of persistent AUB. A systematic review approach is used and a search of the relevant databases from inception to January 20, 2016 was performed.

INITIAL EVALUATION

The initial evaluation begins with a complete history and physical examination followed by appropriate laboratory testing.[12] The initial assessment should exclude pregnancy, evaluate the impact of bleeding on the patient's life, and assess the patient's risks for endometrial cancer and an underlying coagulopathy (**Box 1**).[13]

The history includes age at menarche, menstrual bleeding patterns, heaviness of bleeding (soaking through clothing or bedsheets), pain associated with bleeding, family history of AUB, and signs and symptoms of an underlying coagulopathy.[14] For assessment of the amount of bleeding, the pictorial blood loss assessment chart (PBLAC) is recommended as a validated semiobjective method for assessment of MBL that has been shown to be correlated to MBL measured by alkaline hematin.[15] The use of PBLAC is simple and the chart is easily filled by the patient herself or with the help of the physician (**Fig. 1**).[16,17] In addition to questions related to the amount and pattern of bleeding, specific questions evaluate the patient's risks for endometrial cancer. The American Congress of Obstetricians and Gynecologists recommends endometrial sampling in patients older than the age of 45 with AUB. Patients younger than 45 should have endometrial sampling if they have risk factors for unopposed estrogen, failed medical management, or have a family history of hereditary nonpolyposis colorectal cancer or endometrial cancer.[13] From a coagulopathy risk, one tool commonly used for screening includes questions regarding heavy bleeding since menarche, postpartum hemorrhage, bleeding related to surgery or dental work, family history of bleeding symptoms, frequent bruising, epistaxis, and gum bleeding.[18]

The physical examination should also focus on signs of polycystic ovary syndrome, thyroid disease, and insulin resistance.[12] The physical examination should evaluate for hirsutism, acne, thyroid nodules, acanthosis nigricans, petechiae, ecchymoses, cervical or vaginal lesions, and uterine size. A pelvic examination should be performed to evaluate for uterine size and any structural abnormalities.

Box 1
Initial evaluation of patient presenting with abnormal uterine bleeding

1. Assessment of bleeding:
   a. Acute or chronic?
   b. Pattern:
      i. Regular or irregular bleeding
      ii. Unscheduled bleeding
   c. Amount:
      i. Compared with prior periods
      ii. Presence of blood clots and menstrual accidents
      iii. Other tools for quantification of the amount of bleeding, such as pictorial blood loss assessment chart

2. Assessment of bleeding:
   a. Document change in health-related quality of life
   b. Document patient interest in contraception and future fertility

3. Review medication to detect any iatrogenic causes of abnormal uterine bleeding

4. Screen for coagulopathy using a validated questionnaire[14]: positive screen if
   a. Excessive menstrual bleeding since menarche, or
   b. History of one of the following: postpartum hemorrhage, surgery-related bleeding, or bleeding associated with dental work, or
   c. History of two or more of the following: bruising greater than 5 cm once or twice/month, epistaxis once or twice/month, frequent gum bleeding, family history of bleeding symptoms.

5. Focused physical examination with emphasis on possible causes using the PALM-COEIN classification along with the signs of coagulopathy

6. Perform endometrial biopsy if high risk for endometrial cancer:
   a. Age >45 years
   b. Any of the following condition irrespective of age:
      i. Body mass index >30 kg/m^2
      ii. History of unopposed estrogen use or state
      iii. Tamoxifen
      iv. Family history of endometrial or colon cancer

7. Laboratory tests:
   a. Pregnancy test
   b. Complete blood counts
   c. Coagulopathy laboratory testing if screening was positive
   d. Thyroid-stimulating hormone
   e. Cervical culture
   f. Cervical cytology if indicated per guidelines

The evaluation of patients with risk factors for endometrial cancer includes endometrial sampling. Methods for endometrial sampling include blind methods and sampling under direct visualization. Currently, the most common method for blind endometrial biopsy is the Pipelle (CooperSurgical, Inc, Trumbull, CT). The advantage of this method is that it does not require anesthesia and has a high sensitivity for detection of endometrial cancer, which was estimated in a meta-analysis to be 99.6% in postmenopausal and 91% in premenopausal women.[19] Hysteroscopy allows direct visualization of the uterine cavity and the opportunity for directed biopsy. It is currently the most accurate and precise method for the detection of endometrial polyps and submucosal leiomyomas, which are often overlooked by endometrial biopsy, ultrasonography, or blind curettage. In addition, it can be performed as an outpatient

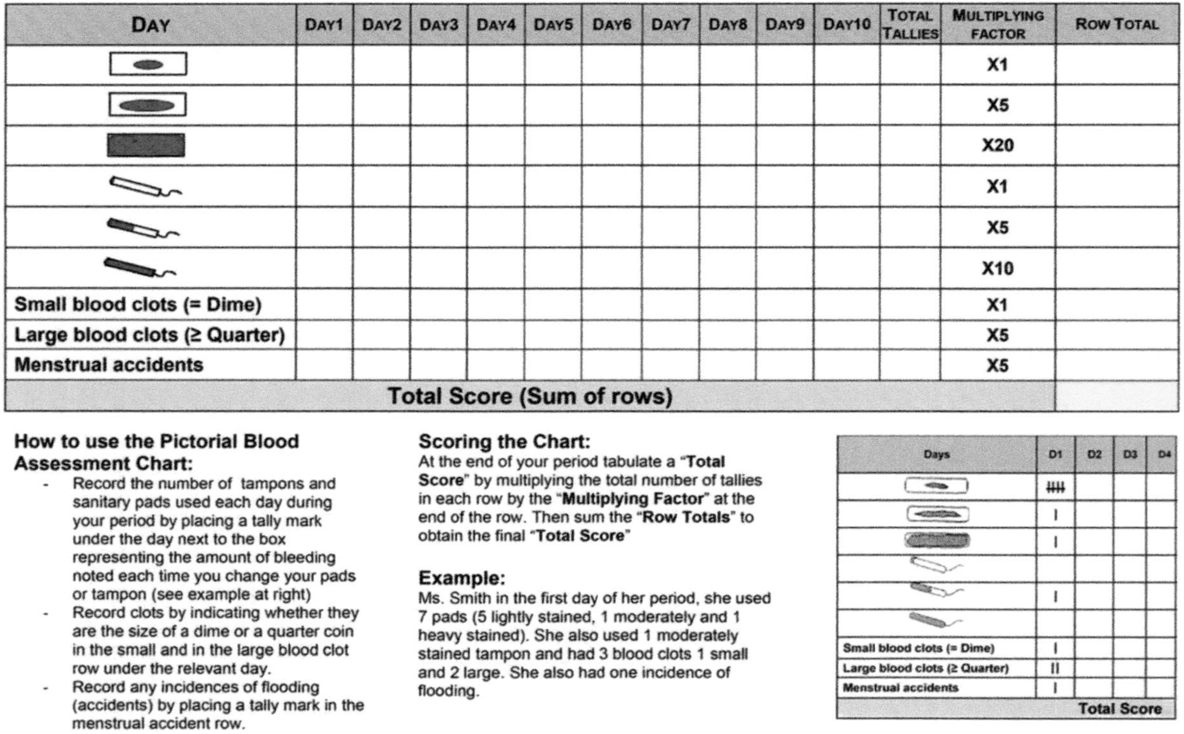

DAY	DAY1	DAY2	DAY3	DAY4	DAY5	DAY6	DAY7	DAY8	DAY9	DAY10	TOTAL TALLIES	MULTIPLYING FACTOR	ROW TOTAL
												X1	
												X5	
												X20	
												X1	
												X5	
												X10	
Small blood clots (= Dime)												X1	
Large blood clots (≥ Quarter)												X5	
Menstrual accidents												X5	
										Total Score (Sum of rows)			

Days	D1	D2	D3	D4
Small blood clots (= Dime)				
Large blood clots (≥ Quarter)				
Menstrual accidents				
				Total Score

How to use the Pictorial Blood Assessment Chart:

- Record the number of tampons and sanitary pads used each day during your period by placing a tally mark under the day next to the box representing the amount of bleeding noted each time you change your pads or tampon (see example at right)
- Record clots by indicating whether they are the size of a dime or a quarter coin in the small and in the large blood clot row under the relevant day.
- Record any incidences of flooding (accidents) by placing a tally mark in the menstrual accident row.

Scoring the Chart:

At the end of your period tabulate a "Total Score" by multiplying the total number of tallies in each row by the "Multiplying Factor" at the end of the row. Then sum the "Row Totals" to obtain the final "Total Score"

Example:

Ms. Smith in the first day of her period, she used 7 pads (5 lightly stained, 1 moderately and 1 heavy stained). She also used 1 moderately stained tampon and had 3 blood clots 1 small and 2 large. She also had one incidence of flooding.

Fig. 1. Pictorial blood loss assessment chart. (*From* El-Nashar SA, Shazly SA, Famuyide AO. Pictorial blood loss assessment chart for quantification of menstrual blood loss: a systematic review. Gynecol Surg 2015; with permission.)

procedure without anesthesia.[20,21] It should be used as a second-line investigation after ultrasound but can be used in the initial evaluation of women with a history of an endometrial polyp or leiomyoma. A flow chart for the initial management and follow-up of AUB is presented in **Fig. 2**.

In patients who are at low risk for endometrial cancer and have a negative screen for coagulopathy, the laboratory evaluation can simply be a pregnancy test, complete blood count, and thyroid-stimulating hormone along with a cervical culture.[13] For patients with a positive coagulopathy screen, further specific testing is needed. Initial testing should include complete blood count with platelet count, prothrombin time, and partial thromboplastin time. Depending on the results of those initial tests further specific testing or referral to hematology should be considered.[13]

INITIAL MEDICAL MANAGEMENT

After a thorough history and physical examination excludes pregnancy, endometrial cancer, an underlying coagulopathy, and an iatrogenic cause of AUB, medical management is the preferred initial treatment. A patient's medical history, bleeding acuity, and contraception desires direct the initial medical management.

Chronic Abnormal Uterine Bleeding

For patients who are stable or those who had successful management of their acute AUB, medical treatment of AUB is indicated. Medical management includes hormonal and nonhormonal options.

Systemic estrogen and progestin
Combined oral contraceptive methods, such as the pill (combined oral contraceptive pill [COCP]) and the ring are effective treatment options for women with AUB caused by anovulation or ovulation dysfunction.[22] They prevent the risks

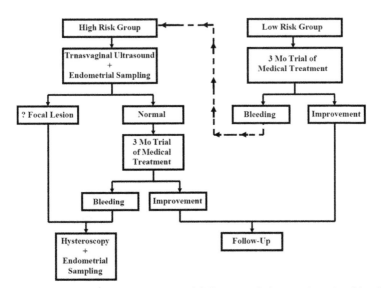

Fig. 2. Flow chart for initial management and follow-up of abnormal uterine bleeding.

associated with prolonged unopposed estrogen stimulation. Extended or continuous use of COCPs has been shown to decrease the number of bleeding episodes per year and decrease heavy menstrual bleeding.[23] A monophasic COCP was compared with mefenamic acid, naproxen, and low-dose danazol. Forty-five women were assigned to each group and the monophasic COCP was shown to be as effective as the other groups in decreasing menstrual bleeding.[24] Furthermore, dienogest/estradiol valerate was compared with a placebo method in a randomized controlled trial and was shown to significantly decrease menstrual bleeding when compared with placebo.[25] Continuous regimens of systemic estrogen and progestin have been compared with cyclic regimens. The continuous regimen had a significant decrease in heavy menstrual bleeding and number of bleeding episodes per year.[26]

Systemic progestin
Women who have contraindications or who cannot tolerate estrogen can use progestin-only methods to decrease their heavy menstrual bleeding. Several different routes and doses of administration are used: continuous systemic administration (daily), cyclic systemic administration (menstrual days 5–21), and continuous local administration.

In women with AUB caused by ovulatory dysfunction, continuous and cyclical administration of a systemic progestin has been shown to be effective in reducing heavy menstrual bleeding and providing excellent cycle control.[27] Commonly used medications include norethindrone acetate (2.5–5 mg daily), medroxyprogesterone acetate (2.5–10 mg daily), micronized progesterone (200–400 mg daily), and megestrol acetate (40–320 mg daily).

Nonhormonal medications
Women who do not desire or have contraindications to hormonal manipulation of AUB can use tranexamic acid or high doses of nonsteroidal anti-inflammatory (NSAIDs). Some NSAIDs have been used to reduce MBL and can be used as nonhormonal treatment, such as mefanemic acid and naproxen. Tranexamic acid is an antifibrinolytic medication that prevents fibrin degradation. Contraindications to tranexamic acid include a history of a thromboembolic event or renal failure. Lukes and colleagues[28] evaluated 115 women with AUB treated with tranexamic acid compared with 72 women treated with placebo. The women who were treated with tranexamic acid had significantly reduced menstrual bleeding and significant improvements in social, professional, and leisure life.

Acute Abnormal Uterine Bleeding
If a patient presents with acute AUB, fluid resuscitation or a blood transfusion may be indicated for initial stabilization. If the patient is unstable and does not respond to volume replacement, surgical intervention must be considered. After stabilization, an evaluation based on the PALM-COEIN system should be initiated. The underlying cause helps guide the management and treatment plan. Medical management is often the initial treatment approach. Multidose regimens of COCPs or intravenous administration of high-dose estrogen is used based on acuity and cause of bleeding. Tranexamic acid and to a lesser extent NSAIDs can be used. If medical treatment is successful then standard management for chronic AUB is recommended. If these medical options are unsuccessful, interventions including hysterectomy and EA are used.[11,13,29]

FOLLOW-UP

Follow-up after initiation of treatment is advised to monitor patient compliance and treatment success. However, there are no data regarding the optimal follow-up interval or its importance. In our practice, we evaluate patients 2 to 3 months after initiating medical treatment. In addition, we found that the use of semiobjective evaluation of MBL, such as PBLAC, or other methods provides the patient and her physician a way of evaluating the reduction of MBL. For example, a patient may present with a PBLAC score of 400, and following treatment it is reduced to 200. This is improved but remains high, and it helps guide counseling and medical decision making. Another important factor is knowledge about the efficacy of different medical treatments. Patients who thoroughly understand the efficacy of treatments are more likely to have successful treatment and increased compliance.

MANAGEMENT OF PERSISTENT ABNORMAL UTERINE BLEEDING

If a patient fails medical management, the treatment options depend on the underlying cause of AUB and her desire for future fertility. In patients with persistent AUB, an evaluation of the endometrial cavity with an ultrasound and endometrial biopsy (if not previously done) is recommended. If a structural abnormality is suspected, a sonohysterography or hysteroscopy is recommended.

If the patient desires future fertility, a repeat trial of medical management or an LNG-IUS can be effective. If the patient does not desire future fertility, an EA should be considered as a less invasive alternative for hysterectomy. Specific treatment options for leiomyomata (AUB-L) are presented elsewhere in this issue (see Laughlin-Tommaso SK: Alternatives to Hysterectomy: Management of Uterine Fibroids, in this issue). Next we summarize the evidence pertaining to the use of LNG-IUS and EA for managing AUB based on the PALM-COEIN classification system.

LEVONORGESTREL INTRAUTERINE SYSTEM

The LNG-IUS is a Food and Drug Administration–approved method of contraception and a medical treatment of heavy menstrual bleeding. It releases 20 μg of progestin daily onto the endometrium, resulting in thinning of the endometrium and thus, decreased blood loss.[30] Although it can be used as an initial treatment, it is also an effective treatment in women with persistent AUB who have failed other medical treatments. It is the only medical treatment that has been compared with a hysterectomy. Because of cost concern, it is often used in patients who have contraindications to systemic hormones, persistent AUB, or those who desire avoidance of surgery.

Levonorgestrel Intrauterine System and Abnormal Uterine Bleeding–PALM

There is limited evidence on the use of LNG-IUS for managing AUB in women with structural abnormalities. For patients with endometrial or cervical polyps (AUB-P), removal of the polyps before insertion of the LNG-IUS is recommended.[31] There is some evidence on the use of LNG-IUS for managing symptoms of pain and bleeding related to adenomyosis (AUB-A). A randomized controlled trial demonstrated that the LNG-IUS was more effective than COCPs in managing pain and bleeding in women with adenomyosis.[31] Another randomized controlled trial evaluated treatment of women with AUB caused by leiomyomas with an LNG-IUS compared with COCPs. The LNG-IUS group had significant improvement of MBL compared with the COCP group.[32] Finally, in some women with endometrial cancer (AUB-M) or hyperplasia who are not candidates for surgical intervention, LNG-IUS is a temporary treatment.[32–41]

Levonorgestrel Intrauterine System and Abnormal Uterine Bleeding–COEIN

For patients with AUB caused by a coagulopathy (AUB-C), the LNG-IUS has been shown to be an effective treatment of heavy menstrual bleeding. Lukes and colleagues[42] demonstrated that the LNG-IUS significantly improves quality of life in these women. Nonetheless, most of the evidence is related to AUB related to the endometrium (AUB-E), ovulatory dysfunction (AUB-O), or causes that are not yet classified (AUB-N). In these patients, there is good evidence to support the effectiveness and safety of LNG-IUS. Several studies have shown a decrease in menstrual bleeding of 86% after 3 months and 97% after 12 months.[43] A multicenter, randomized trial evaluated 571 women with AUB and compared the LNG-IUS with traditional medical management, which included tranexamic acid, mefanamic acid, combined estrogen-progestin, or progestin alone. In the LNG-IUS group, quality of life including social, physical, and emotional well-being was significantly improved.[44] After 2 years, significantly more women continued to use the LNG-IUS compared with the medical management group. An additional randomized controlled trial compared the LNG-IUS with a control group to evaluate if the LNG-IUS could be an alternative treatment to hysterectomy. At 6 months, 64.3% of the patients in the LNG-IUS group cancelled their hysterectomy compared with 14.3% of patient in the control group.[8] Furthermore, a multicenter randomized trial compared 82 patients with AUB treated with an LNG-IUS compared with 83 patients treated with cyclic oral medroxyprogesterone acetate or norethindrone. The LNG-IUS group demonstrated improvements in their bleeding and were more satisfied and continued the treatment.[26]

How to Optimize Levonorgestrel Intrauterine System Outcomes

Although there is strong evidence to support the efficacy and safety of LNG-IUS in treating HMB, there are limited data on the risk factors that affect outcomes after LNG-IUS placement. It is known that early removal of the LNG-IUS is often related to side effects. One of the most common reasons for LNG-IUS removal is spotting in the first 6 months after insertion. This issue is an important target for future research and if there is a prophylactic or treatment strategy to reduce this issue, this will improve use, improve patient satisfaction, and reduce cost associated with early removals.

ENDOMETRIAL ABLATION

A global EA is a minimally invasive surgical alternative for women with persistent AUB who no longer desire fertility. The technique of endometrial destruction was originally developed in 1937. This method used a radiofrequency electrosurgical probe that was blindly inserted into the endometrial cavity. In 1967, cryoendometrial ablation was developed. In the 1980s, more hysteroscopic-guided techniques were introduced including hysteroscopic laser ablation (aluminum based), hysteroscopic resection techniques, and endometrial desiccation. In the 1990s, there was renewed interest in nonresectoscopic ablation techniques and currently, there are five Food and Drug Administration–approved methods: (1) bipolar radiofrequency (NovaSure), (2) hot liquid–filled balloon (ThermaChoice), (3) microwave EA, (4) circulating hot water (Hydro ThermAblator), and (5) cryotherapy (Her Option).

When compared with resectoscopes, the newer nonresectoscope techniques have similar satisfaction rates. The radiofrequency and microwave EA systems had higher amenorrhea rates when compared with the resectoscope technique.[45] A randomized controlled trial compared the NovaSure system with the ThermaChoice system and revealed that Novasure had a significantly greater amenorrhea rate (43%) when compared with ThermaChoice (8%).[46]

An EA is a minimally invasive surgical alternative with the benefits of an outpatient procedure, no abdominal incisions, quicker postoperative recovery, and decreased cost. Indications for global EA include AUB that is unresponsive to the previously discussed medical management. Although not a form of contraception, patients must not desire future fertility because of the concern for abnormal placentation. Patients who are poor surgical candidates or who do not desire a hysterectomy are also candidates for an EA. Contraindications to an EA include pregnancy, active pelvic infection, the presence of an IUS (although this can be removed before ablation), or a known or suspected endometrial hyperplasia or cancer.[47] Relative contraindications include menopause, congenital uterine anomalies, uterine size greater than 10 to 12 cm, and previous transmyometrial uterine surgery including cesarean section or myomectomy. This is because of the concern for a thin myometrium, which may lead to a bladder or bowel injury. There are not sufficient data to suggest that a prior cesarean section may increase the risk of treatment failure. Furthermore, there is no good evidence for a myometrial thickness that is appropriate for an EA.[47]

Before undergoing an EA, a thorough history, physical examination, evaluation of the endometrial cavity, and endometrial sampling should be performed. Transvaginal ultrasound, saline infusion sonohysterography, and hysteroscopy can evaluate uterine length and the presence of intracavitary lesions, such as polyps and submucosal leiomyomas. Endometrial sampling with a biopsy or curettage should be performed on all patients to exclude endometrial hyperplasia and malignancy, which are contraindications to an EA. After this evaluation, the PALM-COEIN system can be used to classify the cause of bleeding and aid in determining the efficacy of an EA.

Endometrial Ablation and Abnormal Uterine Bleeding–Polyp

EAs can be performed on patients with endometrial polyps. There are no randomized controlled trials evaluating a hysteroscopic polypectomy with an EA. Several studies are inconclusive and suggest the presence of endometrial polyps may increase, decrease, or have no influence on EA failure.[48]

Endometrial Ablation and Abnormal Uterine Bleeding–Adenomyosis

Adenomyosis commonly presents with heavy menstrual bleeding and pelvic pain. El-Nashar and colleagues[10] demonstrated that preoperative severe dysmenorrhea is a significant predictor of EA failure. There are limited data evaluating the effects of an EA on suspected or unsuspected adenomyosis. A prospective study evaluated 213 patients who underwent a Novasure EA and found that 22 (10.3%) underwent a hysterectomy because of a failed procedure. Of the 22 patients, 10 (45.5%) were found to have adenomyosis in the hysterectomy specimen. Deep adenomyosis (>2.5 mm endometrial penetration) was associated with a higher failure rate.[49] Recently our group evaluated the combined use of a LNG-IUS and an EA in patients with preoperative dysmenorrhea. In this work, we compared women who had an LNG-IUS inserted at the time of EA with a control group of women who only underwent an EA. Sonographic signs of adenomyosis were often seen in the EA/LNG-IUS group. There were two treatment failures in the EA/LNG-IUS group; however, none of the patients went on to have a hysterectomy. The control group had 19 treatment failures and 16 went on to have a hysterectomy.[50] The combination of an EA/LNG-IUS may be a feasible option for patients with dysmenorrhea caused by adenomyosis who undergo an EA to decrease failure rates.

The association between adenomyosis and treatment failure after EA is controversial. Carey and colleagues[51] performed a retrospective analysis of 69 hysterectomy specimens of patients who failed an EA. The most common reasons for undergoing a hysterectomy was bleeding (51%), pain (28%), and bleeding and pain (19%). The most common pathologic finding was leiomyoma in the patients who underwent an EA for bleeding, whereas hematometra was found in 26% of patients who underwent an EA because of pain. This finding was different than those reported previously about the association of failure with the presence of undiagnosed adenomyosis.

Endometrial Ablation and Abnormal Uterine Bleeding–Leiomyoma

Submucosal leiomyomas most often contribute to AUB. Although Wishall and colleagues[9] identified that leiomyomas may quadruple the risk for failed EA and subsequent hysterectomy, many studies suggest that leiomyoma may be hysteroscopically resected before an EA with good outcomes. Loffer[52] evaluated the effect of a hysteroscopic resection of submucosal leiomyomas performed at the same time of an EA. The author compared 104 patients who underwent a hysteroscopic myomectomy without an EA with 73 patients who underwent a hysteroscopic myomectomy with an EA. Bleeding significantly decreased in the group who had an EA versus the group that did not (95.9% vs 80.8%; $P = .003$). Loffer[52] suggested that complete excision of the myoma with an EA improved results. Subsequent hysterectomy rates were not decreased in the EA. Furthermore, Sabbah and Desaulniers[53] evaluated 65 women who underwent an EA because of AUB caused by type I and II submucosal myomas up to 3 cm with and without polyps over 12 months. The NovaSure system reduced uterine blood loss successfully in 95% of patients and induced amenorrhea in 69% of patients.

Endometrial Ablation and Abnormal Uterine Bleeding–Coagulopathy

Women diagnosed with coagulopathies caused by congenital or acquired bleeding disorders (von Willebrand disease, inherited bleeding disorders, thrombocytopenia, and abnormal platelet function) often present with AUB. Often times, these women are on long-term anticoagulation, which can cause AUB. El-Nashar and colleagues[11] evaluated the efficacy of EA in this patient population. The authors compared 41 patients with a bleeding disorder who underwent an EA with 111 patients without a bleeding disorder who underwent an EA. There were no differences in bleeding patterns, complications, subsequent hysterectomies, or time to treatment failure between the groups, suggesting an EA is an effective alternative treatment in women with AUB caused by coagulation disorders.

Endometrial Ablation and Abnormal Uterine Bleeding–Ovulatory Dysfunction

AUB caused by an ovulatory dysfunction is defined as irregular, heavy bleeding when other causes have been excluded. This patient population is typically excluded as candidates for an EA given the concern for future development of an endometrial hyperplasia or malignancy. Hokenstad and colleagues[54] performed a retrospective cohort study evaluating the efficacy and safety of an EA for the treatment of AUB caused by an ovulatory dysfunction. The authors compared rates of amenorrhea and treatment failure after 5 years of 169 patients with AUB-O with 320 patients with AUB-E. The rates of amenorrhea and treatment failure were similar between the two groups (11.8% vs 13.8% and 11.7% vs 12.3%). There were no endometrial cancers after EA in the AUB-O group.

On the contrary, a systematic review evaluated the number of endometrial cancer cases after an EA, which found 22 cases and most were stage I at diagnosis. The interval to detection was 2 weeks to 10 years. Most of the patients did have risk factors for endometrial cancer.[55]

Madsen and colleagues[56] performed a retrospective analysis of 263 obese (body mass index >30) and 403 nonobese patients who underwent an EA. There were no significant differences in treatment failures or adverse events between the two groups, suggesting an EA can be an alternative to hysterectomy to avoid the morbidities associated with hysterectomy in the obese population.

Endometrial Ablation and Abnormal Uterine Bleeding–Endometrial

An EA is most effective when AUB is caused by a primary endometrial dysfunction. A randomized trial compared the 5-year follow-up of medical management use with an EA. After 5 years, 10% of the patients receiving medical management continued this therapy, whereas 77% of these patients underwent surgical intervention. In the EA group, 27% underwent further surgical intervention, of which 18% were a hysterectomy. The EA group had higher satisfaction rates and improvement in their health-related quality of life.[45] A Cochrane meta-analysis compared the LNG-IUS with an EA. After 1 year, both treatments had similar satisfaction rates and improvements in

Table 1
Risk factors known or suspected to be related to treatment failure after endometrial ablation

Treatment Outcome	Risk Factor	Results (Number of Studies)	References
Need for hysterectomy after ablation	Age <45	Increased risk (2)	10
	Parity ≥5	Increased risk (1)	10
	Dysmenorrhea	Increased risk (1)	10
	Tubal ligation	Increased risk (1)	10
	C-section	Increased risk (1), no effect (2)	9,10,57
	BMI >30 kg/m^2	Increased risk (1)	56
	Irregular bleeding	No effect (1)	54
	RFA vs TBA	No effect (3)	46,58,59
	Coagulopathy	No effect (2)	25
	High-risk surgical patients	No effect (1)	—
	Procedure not done in the OR	Increased risk (1)	9
	Uterine abnormalities on imaging, including leiomyoma, adenomyosis, thickened endometrial strip, and polyps	Increased risk (1), no effect (1)	9
	Larger uterine size	Increased risk (1)	60
	Less time with RFA	Increased risk (1)	60
Amenorrhea after ablation	Age >45	Increased risk (1)	10
	Uterine length <9 cm	Increased risk (1)	10
	Endometrial thickness <4 mm	Increased risk (1)	10
	RFA compared with TBA	Increased risk (1)	46,58,59
Pain after ablation	Dysmenorrhea	Increased risk (1)	9
	Tubal sterilization	Increased risk (1)	9

Abbreviations: BMI, body mass index; OR, operative room; RFA, radiofrequency ablation; TBA, thermal balloon ablation.

quality of life. The EA controlled bleeding patterns better after 1 year; however, after 2 and 3 years, both interventions were comparable.

How to Optimize Outcomes After Endometrial Ablation

Compared with a hysterectomy, global EA initially has similar efficacy with lower costs and complication rates. However, after 4 to 5 years, 30% of patients have a hysterectomy because of persistent bleeding or pain.[5] Failure of an EA is often defined as a repeat EA or subsequent hysterectomy. El-Nashar and colleagues[10] evaluated amenorrhea and failure rates in 816 women who underwent an EA. The amenorrhea rate (no menses 12 months after EA) was 23% and the 5-year failure rate (defined as reablation or subsequent hysterectomy) was 16%. Predictors of amenorrhea included age 45 years or older, uterine length less than 9 cm, and an endometrial thickness less than 4 mm. Amenorrhea rates were higher if the radiofrequency EA system was used compared with the thermal balloon ablation system. Predictors of treatment failure were age younger than 45 years, parity of five or more, prior tubal ligation, and preoperative history of dysmenorrhea. This study evaluated many risk factors for amenorrhea and treatment failure. The current knowledge on risk factors is summarized in **Table 1**.

To decrease the failure of an EA, proper patient selection and counseling is crucial. To optimize outcomes, risk factors for failure should be identified. This allows for optimal selection of patients who will benefit from an EA, which facilitates successful treatment, decreases the need for additional surgery, increases patient satisfaction, and possibly reduces cost (**Fig. 3**). This process can be applied to all AUB treatments

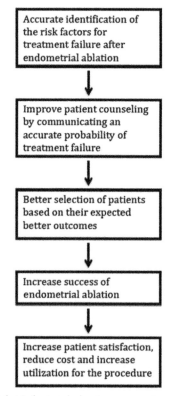

Fig. 3. How identification of risk factors helps improve outcomes after ablation.

to help improve outcomes, which may ultimately increase patient satisfaction and avoid hysterectomy.

SUMMARY

AUB is a common problem that significantly impacts a patient's quality of life. Assessment of cancer risk (AUB-M), bleeding related to coagulopathy (AUB-C), and bleeding related to medications (AUB-I) are recommended before initiating medical treatment. Initial treatment includes hormonal and nonhormonal options, such as COCPs, oral progestins, tranexamic acid, and NSAIDs. If initial management fails, a thorough evaluation for structural abnormalities and other components of PALM-COEIN system is needed. If there are no structural abnormalities identified, a repeat trial of medical treatment or more effective treatments including LNG-IUS or EA can be used based on patient preferences and fertility wishes. Both LNG-IUS and EA are effective, less invasive, and safe alternatives to hysterectomy for women with AUB-E and AUB-N and for selected patients with AUB-O. A hysterectomy remains the definitive treatment of AUB regardless of the suspected cause when alternative treatments fail. Future studies should focus on the identification of risk factors associated with treatment outcomes, which will better facilitate patient counseling, patient selection for treatment modalities, and ultimately may improve patient satisfaction and reduce cost.

REFERENCES

1. Liu Z, Doan QV, Blumenthal P, et al. A systematic review evaluating health-related quality of life, work impairment, and health-care costs and utilization in abnormal uterine bleeding. Value Health 2007;10(3):183–94.
2. Fraser IS, Langham S, Uhl-Hochgraeber K. Health-related quality of life and economic burden of abnormal uterine bleeding. Obstet Gynecol 4:179–89.
3. Munro MG, Critchley HO, Broder MS, et al. FIGO classification system (PALM-COEIN) for causes of abnormal uterine bleeding in nongravid women of reproductive age. Int J Gynaecol Obstet 2011;113(1):3–13.
4. ACOG criteria set. Hysterectomy, abdominal or vaginal for abnormal uterine bleeding. Number 28, November 1997. Committee on Quality Assessment. American College of Obstetricians and Gynecologists. Int J Gynaecol Obstet 1998;60(3):314–5.
5. Dickersin K, Munro MG, Clark M, et al. Hysterectomy compared with endometrial ablation for dysfunctional uterine bleeding: a randomized controlled trial. Obstet Gynecol 2007;110(6):1279–89.
6. Hurskainen R, Teperi J, Rissanen P, et al. Quality of life and cost-effectiveness of levonorgestrel-releasing intrauterine system versus hysterectomy for treatment of menorrhagia: a randomised trial. Lancet 2001;357(9252):273–7.
7. Hurskainen R, Teperi J, Rissanen P, et al. Clinical outcomes and costs with the levonorgestrel-releasing intrauterine system or hysterectomy for treatment of menorrhagia: randomized trial 5-year follow-up. JAMA 2004;291(12):1456–63.
8. Lahteenmaki P, Haukkamaa M, Puolakka J, et al. Open randomised study of use of levonorgestrel releasing intrauterine system as alternative to hysterectomy. BMJ 1998;316(7138):1122–6.
9. Wishall KM, Price J, Pereira N, et al. Postablation risk factors for pain and subsequent hysterectomy. Obstet Gynecol 2014;124(5):904–10.
10. El-Nashar SA, Hopkins MR, Creedon DJ, et al. Prediction of treatment outcomes after global endometrial ablation. Obstet Gynecol 2009;113(1):97–106.

11. El-Nashar SA, Hopkins MR, Feitoza SS, et al. Global endometrial ablation for menorrhagia in women with bleeding disorders. Obstet Gynecol 2007;109(6): 1381–7.
12. Committee on Practice Bulletins—Gynecology. Practice bulletin No. 128: diagnosis of abnormal uterine bleeding in reproductive-aged women. Obstet Gynecol 2012;120(1):197–206.
13. ACOG committee opinion No. 557: Management of acute abnormal uterine bleeding in nonpregnant reproductive-aged women. Obstet Gynecol 2013; 121(4):891–6.
14. Kouides PA, Conard J, Peyvandi F, et al. Hemostasis and menstruation: appropriate investigation for underlying disorders of hemostasis in women with excessive menstrual bleeding. Fertil Steril 2005;84(5):1345–51.
15. Zakherah MS, Sayed GH, El-Nashar SA, et al. Pictorial blood loss assessment chart in the evaluation of heavy menstrual bleeding: diagnostic accuracy compared to alkaline hematin. Gynecol Obstet Invest 2011;71(4):281–4.
16. Higham JM, O'Brien PM, Shaw RW. Assessment of menstrual blood loss using a pictorial chart. Br J Obstet Gynaecol 1990;97(8):734–9.
17. El-Nashar SA, Shazly SA, Famuyide AO. Pictorial blood loss assessment chart for quantification of menstrual blood loss: a systematic review. Gynecol Surg 2015.
18. Kadir RA, Lukes AS, Kouides PA, et al. Management of excessive menstrual bleeding in women with hemostatic disorders. Fertil Steril 2005;84(5):1352–9.
19. Dijkhuizen FP, Lukes AS, Kouides PA, et al. The accuracy of endometrial sampling in the diagnosis of patients with endometrial carcinoma and hyperplasia: a meta-analysis. Cancer 2000;89(8):1765–72.
20. Bain C, Parkin DE, Cooper KG. Is outpatient diagnostic hysteroscopy more useful than endometrial biopsy alone for the investigation of abnormal uterine bleeding in unselected premenopausal women? A randomised comparison. BJOG 2002; 109(7):805–11.
21. Bain C, Cooper KG, Parkin DE. Microwave endometrial ablation versus endometrial resection: a randomized controlled trial. Obstet Gynecol 2002;99(6):983–7.
22. Kaunitz AM, Burkman RT, Fisher AC, et al. Cycle control with a 21-day compared with a 24-day oral contraceptive pill: a randomized controlled trial. Obstet Gynecol 2009;114(6):1205–12.
23. Anderson FD, Hait H. A multicenter, randomized study of an extended cycle oral contraceptive. Contraception 2003;68(2):89–96.
24. Fraser IS, McCarron G. Randomized trial of 2 hormonal and 2 prostaglandin-inhibiting agents in women with a complaint of menorrhagia. Aust N Z J Obstet Gynaecol 1991;31(1):66–70.
25. Braunstein JB, Hausfeld J, Hausfeld J, et al. Economics of reducing menstruation with trimonthly-cycle oral contraceptive therapy: comparison with standard-cycle regimens. Obstet Gynecol 2003;102(4):699–708.
26. Kaunitz AM, Portman DJ, Hait H, et al. Adding low-dose estrogen to the hormone-free interval: impact on bleeding patterns in users of a 91-day extended regimen oral contraceptive. Contraception 2009;79(5):350–5.
27. Hickey M, Higham JM, Fraser I. Progestogens with or without oestrogen for irregular uterine bleeding associated with anovulation. Cochrane Database Syst Rev 2012;(9):CD001895.
28. Lukes AS, Moore KA, Muse KN, et al. Tranexamic acid treatment for heavy menstrual bleeding: a randomized controlled trial. Obstet Gynecol 2010;116(4): 865–75.

29. El-Nashar SA, Hopkins MR, Barnes SA, et al. Health-related quality of life and patient satisfaction after global endometrial ablation for menorrhagia in women with bleeding disorders: a follow-up survey and systematic review. Am J Obstet Gynecol 2010;202(4):348.e1–7.
30. Sayed GH, Zakherah MS, El-Nashar SA, et al. A randomized clinical trial of a levonorgestrel-releasing intrauterine system and a low-dose combined oral contraceptive for fibroid-related menorrhagia. Int J Gynaecol Obstet 2011;112(2):126–30.
31. Henriquez DD, van Dongen H, Wolterbeek R, et al. Polypectomy in premenopausal women with abnormal uterine bleeding: effectiveness of hysteroscopic removal. J Minim Invasive Gynecol 2007;14(1):59–63.
32. Fambrini M, Bargelli G, Peruzzi E, et al. Levonorgestrel-releasing intrauterine system alone as primary treatment in young women with early endometrial cancer: case report. J Minim Invasive Gynecol 2009;16(5):630–3.
33. Kim MK, Yoon BS, Park H, et al. Conservative treatment with medroxyprogesterone acetate plus levonorgestrel intrauterine system for early-stage endometrial cancer in young women: pilot study. Int J Gynecol Cancer 2011;21(4):673–7.
34. Kim MK, Seong SJ, Lee TS, et al. Treatment with medroxyprogesterone acetate plus levonorgestrel-releasing intrauterine system for early-stage endometrial cancer in young women: single-arm, prospective multicenter study: Korean Gynecologic Oncology Group study (KGOG2009). Jpn J Clin Oncol 2012;42(12):1215–8.
35. Pashov AI, Tskhay VB, Ionouchene SV. The combined GnRH-agonist and intrauterine levonorgestrel-releasing system treatment of complicated atypical hyperplasia and endometrial cancer: a pilot study. Gynecol Endocrinol 2012;28(7):559–61.
36. Kim MK, Seong SJ, Kim YS, et al. Combined medroxyprogesterone acetate/levonorgestrel-intrauterine system treatment in young women with early-stage endometrial cancer. Am J Obstet Gynecol 2013;209(4):358.e1–4.
37. Morelli M, Di Cello A, Venturella R, et al. Efficacy of the levonorgestrel intrauterine system (LNG-IUS) in the prevention of the atypical endometrial hyperplasia and endometrial cancer: retrospective data from selected obese menopausal symptomatic women. Gynecol Endocrinol 2013;29(2):156–9.
38. Fu Y, Zhuang Z. Long-term effects of levonorgestrel-releasing intrauterine system on tamoxifen-treated breast cancer patients: a meta-analysis. Int J Clin Exp Pathol 2014;7(10):6419–29.
39. Shi Q, Li J, Li M, et al. The role of levonorgestrel-releasing intrauterine system for endometrial protection in women with breast cancer taking tamoxifen. Eur J Gynaecol Oncol 2014;35(5):492–8.
40. Soini T, Hurskainen R, Grénman S, et al. Cancer risk in women using the levonorgestrel-releasing intrauterine system in Finland. Obstet Gynecol 2014;124(2 Pt 1):292–9.
41. Dominick S, Hickey M, Chin J, et al. Levonorgestrel intrauterine system for endometrial protection in women with breast cancer on adjuvant tamoxifen. Cochrane Database Syst Rev 2015;(12):CD007245.
42. Lukes AS, Reardon B, Arepally G. Use of the levonorgestrel-releasing intrauterine system in women with hemostatic disorders. Fertil Steril 2008;90(3):673–7.
43. Lethaby AE, Cooke I, Rees M. Progesterone or progestogen-releasing intrauterine systems for heavy menstrual bleeding. Cochrane Database Syst Rev 2005;(4):CD002126.
44. Gupta J, Kai J, Middleton L, et al. Levonorgestrel intrauterine system versus medical therapy for menorrhagia. N Engl J Med 2013;368(2):128–37.

45. Cooper JM, Anderson TL, Fortin CA, et al. Microwave endometrial ablation vs. rollerball electroablation for menorrhagia: a multicenter randomized trial. J Am Assoc Gynecol Laparosc 2004;11(3):394–403.
46. Bongers MY, Bourdrez P, Mol BW, et al. Randomised controlled trial of bipolar radio-frequency endometrial ablation and balloon endometrial ablation. BJOG 2004;111(10):1095–102.
47. American College of Obstetrician and Gynecologists, ACOG Practice Bulletins. List of titles December 2007. Obstet Gynecol 2007;110(6):1469–71.
48. Tjarks M, Van Voorhis BJ. Treatment of endometrial polyps. Obstet Gynecol 2000; 96(6):886–9.
49. Mengerink BB, van der Wurff AA, ter Haar JF, et al. Effect of undiagnosed deep adenomyosis after failed NovaSure endometrial ablation. J Minim Invasive Gynecol 2015;22(2):239–44.
50. Papadakis EP, El-Nashar SA, Laughlin-Tommaso SK, et al. Combined endometrial ablation and levonorgestrel intrauterine system use in women with dysmenorrhea and heavy menstrual bleeding: novel approach for challenging cases. J Minim Invasive Gynecol 2015;22(7):1203–7.
51. Carey ET, El-Nashar SA, Hopkins MR, et al. Pathologic characteristics of hysterectomy specimens in women undergoing hysterectomy after global endometrial ablation. J Minim Invasive Gynecol 2011;18(1):96–9.
52. Loffer FD. Endometrial ablation in patients with myomas. Curr Opin Obstet Gynecol 2006;18(4):391–3.
53. Sabbah R, Desaulniers G. Use of the NovaSure Impedance Controlled Endometrial Ablation System in patients with intracavitary disease: 12-month follow-up results of a prospective, single-arm clinical study. J Minim Invasive Gynecol 2006;13(5):467–71.
54. Hokenstad AN, El-Nashar SA, Khan Z, et al. Endometrial ablation in women with abnormal uterine bleeding related to ovulatory dysfunction: a cohort study. J Minim Invasive Gynecol 2015;22(7):1225–30.
55. AlHilli MM, Hopkins MR, Famuyide AO. Endometrial cancer after endometrial ablation: systematic review of medical literature. J Minim Invasive Gynecol 2011;18(3):393–400.
56. Madsen AM, El-Nashar SA, Hopkins MR, et al. Endometrial ablation for the treatment of heavy menstrual bleeding in obese women. Int J Gynaecol Obstet 2013; 121(1):20–3.
57. Khan Z, El-Nashar SA, Hopkins MR, et al. Efficacy and safety of global endometrial ablation after cesarean delivery: a cohort study. Am J Obstet Gynecol 2011; 205(5):450.e1–4.
58. Abbott J, Hawe J, Hunter D, et al. A double-blind randomized trial comparing the Cavaterm and the NovaSure endometrial ablation systems for the treatment of dysfunctional uterine bleeding. Fertil Steril 2003;80(1):203–8.
59. El-Nashar SA, Hopkins MR, Creedon DJ, et al. Efficacy of bipolar radiofrequency endometrial ablation vs thermal balloon ablation for management of menorrhagia: a population-based cohort. J Minim Invasive Gynecol 2009;16(6):692–9.
60. Shazly SA, Famuyide AO, El-Nashar SA, et al. Intraoperative predictors of long-term outcomes after radiofrequency endometrial ablation. J Minim Invasive Gynecol 2016;23(4):582–9.

Hysterectomy for Benign Conditions of the Uterus

Total Abdominal Hysterectomy

Michael Moen, MD*

KEYWORDS

- Abdominal hysterectomy • Surgical technique • Preoperative evaluation
- Postoperative care

KEY POINTS

- Regardless of increasing use of minimally invasive hysterectomy techniques, a certain percentage of hysterectomies will require an open abdominal approach, most commonly due to large uterine fibroids, large ovarian masses, and extensive pelvic adhesive disease such as occurs with advanced stages of endometriosis.
- The basic surgical technique for abdominal hysterectomy has remained relatively unchanged for several decades and key steps include retroperitoneal dissection with identification of the ureters, sharp dissection of the bladder from the lower uterine segment and cervix, and isolation and control of the uterine vessels.
- Standardized approaches for patient evaluation, preoperative preparation, and postoperative care can reduce morbidity and enhance patient recovery with abdominal hysterectomy.

HISTORICAL PERSPECTIVE

Credit for the first abdominal hysterectomy with a surviving patient goes to Walter Burnham of Lowell, Massachusetts, who performed the operation in 1853. Burnham believed he was operating on a large ovarian cyst but instead encountered a large fibroid uterus. Ether was used for anesthesia and caused the patient to vomit, resulting in extrusion of the myomatous uterus through the incision. Burnham was unable to replace the myoma and proceeded with ligation of both uterine arteries and a supracervical hysterectomy. The patient recovered and Burnham performed 15 additional hysterectomies over the following 13 years; however, only 3 of these patients survived with the others dying of sepsis, peritonitis, or hemorrhage.

Obstetrics and Gynecology, Chicago Medical School, Rosalind Franklin University, 3333 Green Bay Road, North Chicago, IL 60064, USA
* Corresponding author. 1875 Dempster Street, Suite 665, Park Ridge, IL 60068.
E-mail address: michael.moen@advocatehealth.com

Obstet Gynecol Clin N Am 43 (2016) 431–440
http://dx.doi.org/10.1016/j.ogc.2016.04.003
0889-8545/16/$ – see front matter © 2016 Elsevier Inc. All rights reserved.
obgyn.theclinics.com

CURRENT TRENDS

Today, hysterectomy is currently the most frequently performed major gynecologic surgical procedure with more than 400,000 cases performed annually in the United States.[1] With the introduction of laparoscopic assistance and, more recently, robotic assistance, current approaches for hysterectomy allow minimally invasive techniques and have resulted in lower morbidity. Despite the increasing use of minimally invasive techniques, the open abdominal approach remains the most common technique used, accounting for more than 50% of all hysterectomies.[1] Some investigators have pointed out the need to decrease open cases by increasing the use of minimally invasive techniques, and rates of abdominal hysterectomy as low as 35% have been demonstrated.[2,3] Regardless of the increasing performance of minimally invasive techniques, a certain percentage of hysterectomies will require an open abdominal approach. Common indications for hysterectomy include abnormal uterine bleeding, uterine fibroids, pelvic pain, and pelvic organ prolapse. Indications for the abdominal approach to hysterectomy include large fibroids, large ovarian cysts, and dense adhesive disease, often seen with advanced endometriosis and pelvic inflammatory disease.

PREOPERATIVE PREPARATION

Documentation of surgical planning and informed consent are critical components of the preoperative evaluation. **Box 1** lists factors to consider before hysterectomy.[4] Prophylactic antibiotics have been shown to reduce infectious complications after abdominal hysterectomy. A single intravenous dose of first-generation cephalosporin given within 30 minutes of incision time is used. Women undergoing hysterectomy require thromboprophylaxis. In most cases, intermittent pneumatic compression is sufficient for this purpose.[5] Patients receiving chronic antithrombotic therapy are at risk of perioperative bleeding and guidelines for management of these patients are available.[6] Although some centers continue to perform bowel preparation before abdominal surgery, recent data suggests routine bowel preparation is not necessary.[7]

SURGICAL TECHNIQUE

The basic steps for abdominal hysterectomy are listed in **Box 2**. After anesthesia has been achieved, the patient is placed in a frog-leg position and examination under

---

Box 1
Preoperative evaluation and documentation before hysterectomy

Informed consent: options, risks, benefits, goals of treatment, and expected outcomes

Documentation of completion of childbearing

Documentation that an adequate trial of medical or nonsurgical management has been offered and attempted or refused

Documentation of risks and benefits of prophylactic oophorectomy or salpingectomy

Evaluation of health status and determination if medical consultation is needed

Evaluation for preoperative anemia requiring correction

Review most recent cervical cytology and need for other gynecologic investigation, such as endometrial assessment

Adapted from Falcone T, Walters M. Hysterectomy for benign disease. Obstet Gynecol 2008;111:755; with permission.

Box 2
Basic steps for abdominal hysterectomy

1. Patient positioning, examination under anesthesia, sterile preparation, and draping

2. Incision, placement of self-retaining retractor, adhesiolysis (if needed), packing of the bowel

3. Round ligament transection, retroperitoneal dissection with identification of ureter

4. Control of utero-ovarian vessels or infundibulopelvic ligament (if adnexa is to be removed)

5. Incision of anterior peritoneum and dissection of bladder from cervix

6. Isolation and control of uterine vessels

7. Clamping and cutting of parametrial tissues along cervix

8. Incision into upper vagina and removal of specimen

9. Closure of vaginal cuff

10. Final inspection and closure of incision

---

anesthesia is performed. The vagina is prepped with sterile solution, a Foley catheter is placed, and the patient is returned to the supine position. The abdomen is prepped with a sterile solution and surgical drapes are placed. The surgical time-out is then performed.

Choice of incision depends on expected pathologic condition. For a smaller uterus, a transverse incision, such as the Pfannenstiel incision, can be used. In cases in which the uterus is large or extensive disease extending beyond the uterus, such as endometriosis or adhesions, is suspected, a vertical midline incision is used. After the incision is made and the peritoneal cavity entered, a survey of the abdomen and pelvis is conducted and, if needed, lysis of abdominal wall, omental, and bowel adhesions is performed. A self-retaining retractor is placed in the incision. Common retractors include the Balfour, O'Connor-O'Sullivan, and the Bookwalter. Recently, soft, self-retaining retractors, such as the Alexis, have been introduced and can be used. Once the retractor is placed, the bowel is packed away from the operative field using moist lap sponges. In cases of very large masses, the mass might need to be delivered before placing the retractor and packing the bowel.

The uterus is then grasped with clamps placed across the proximal round ligament, Fallopian tube, and utero-ovarian ligament. Traction is then applied, moving the uterus to one side, and the surgeon begins the hysterectomy by clamping and transecting the round ligament (**Fig. 1**). Transecting the round ligament allows access to the retroperitoneal space. The peritoneal incision is extended posteriorly, being careful to incise parallel to the ovarian vessels and not toward them. The ureter is identified as it crosses the bifurcation of the common iliac artery and can be followed through its course into the pelvis along the medial leaf of the broad ligament (**Fig. 2**). With the ureter in view, the peritoneum of the medial leaf of the broad ligament is perforated between the ureter and the ovarian vessels (**Fig. 3**). If the adnexa are to be removed, the infundibulopelvic ligament with the contained ovarian vessels is clamped, cut, and ligated. If the adnexa are to remain, then the utero-ovarian ligament is clamped, cut, and ligated distal to the adnexa. The most common method used to control this pedicle is to first place a free tie and then a suture ligature. The same procedure is then performed on the opposite side.

After controlling the ovarian vasculature on each side, the anterior peritoneum is incised (**Fig. 4**). If a previous cesarean section scar is present, it is best to make the

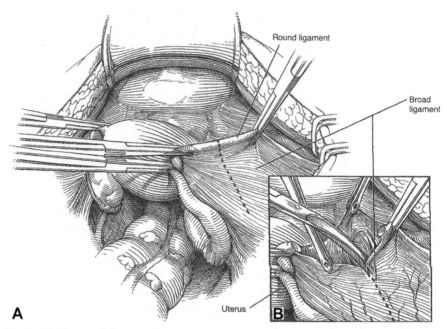

Fig. 1. (*A*) The round ligament is transected to expose the retroperitoneal space. (*B*) Posterior extension of the peritoneal incision parallel to the ovarian vessels. (*From* Lee RA. Atlas of gynecologic surgery. Philadelphia: W.B. Saunders; 1992. Used with permission of Mayo Foundation for Medical Education and Research. All rights reserved.)

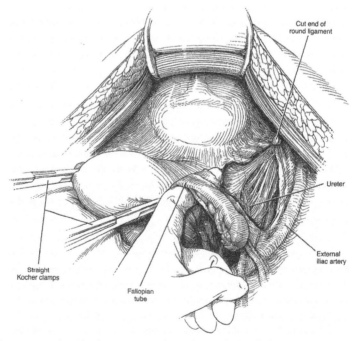

Fig. 2. The ureter is identified in its course along the medial leaf of the broad ligament. (*From* Lee RA. Atlas of gynecologic surgery. Philadelphia: W.B. Saunders; 1992. Used with permission of Mayo Foundation for Medical Education and Research. All rights reserved.)

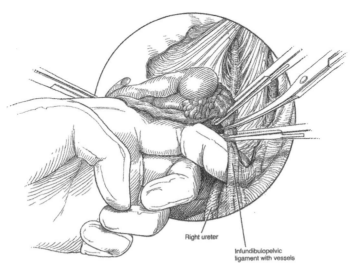

Fig. 3. The peritoneum of the medial leaf of the broad ligament is perforated to isolate the infundibulopelvic ligament, which is then clamped, cut, and tied. (*From* Lee RA. Atlas of gynecologic surgery. Philadelphia: W.B. Saunders; 1992. Used with permission of Mayo Foundation for Medical Education and Research. All rights reserved.)

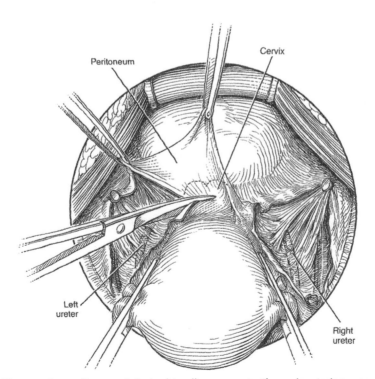

Fig. 4. The anterior peritoneum is incised to allow access to the vesicouterine space. (*From* Lee RA. Atlas of gynecologic surgery. Philadelphia: W.B. Saunders; 1992. Used with permission of Mayo Foundation for Medical Education and Research. All rights reserved.)

peritoneal incision below the scar to gain access to the avascular areolar tissue between the bladder and cervix. Sharp dissection is performed to dissect the bladder from the lower uterine segment and cervix (**Fig. 5**).

In cases of distorted anatomy, such as severe endometriosis, it is helpful to develop the paravesical and pararectal spaces. The paravesical space is an avascular space lateral to the bladder and anterior to the cardinal ligament. Its lateral border is the external iliac vessels. The pararectal space is posterior to the cardinal ligament and lateral to the rectum. It can be developed by gentle blunt dissection between the ureter and internal iliac vessels. When necessary, the rectum can be dissected from the cervix by incising the peritoneum between the uterosacral ligaments, which allows access to the avascular space between the rectum and cervix.

The uterine vessels are exposed by removing loose connective tissue around the vessels (skeletonizing). With the bladder mobilized anteriorly and the ureter laterally, the uterine vessels can be safely clamped. Common techniques include clamping perpendicular to the uterine vessels with a curved Heaney clamp or clamping diagonally across the cardinal ligament with a Kocher clamp (**Fig. 6**). Once the uterine vessels have been clamped, cut, and sutured, successive bites of the remaining parametrial tissue are taken using straight clamps placed along the lateral edge of the cervix. The parametrial tissue is progressively clamped, cut, and ligated until the upper vagina is reached. Curved clamps are used again to clamp the uterosacral ligaments, which are then transected and tied.

At this point, the vagina is entered with scissors and a circumferential incision is made, separating the uterus and cervix from the upper vagina. The corners of the

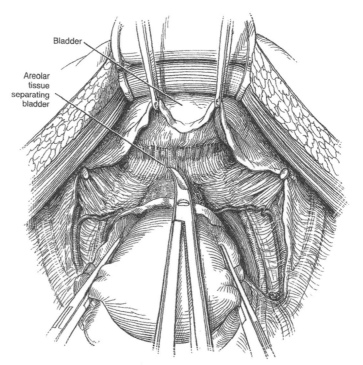

Fig. 5. Sharp dissection is used to separate the bladder from the lower uterine segment and cervix. (*From* Lee RA. Atlas of gynecologic surgery. Philadelphia: W.B. Saunders; 1992. Used with permission of Mayo Foundation for Medical Education and Research. All rights reserved.)

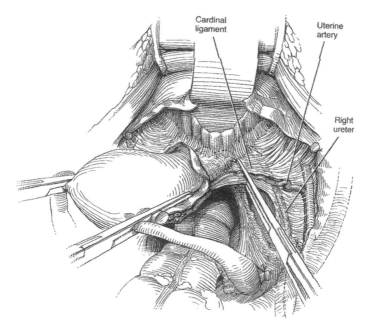

Fig. 6. The uterine vessels are clamped placing the tip of the clamp against the cervix. (*From* Lee RA. Atlas of gynecologic surgery. Philadelphia: W.B. Saunders; 1992. Used with permission of Mayo Foundation for Medical Education and Research. All rights reserved.)

vaginal cuff are grasped and cuff is sutured closed, typically using figure-8 or running sutures (**Fig. 7**). If a supracervical hysterectomy is planned, the parametrial tissues are clamped and cut to the level of the midcervix and the cervix is then transected. Cautery can be used for this step. The endocervix can be resected or cauterized and the stump closed with suture. The stump can also be covered with peritoneum.

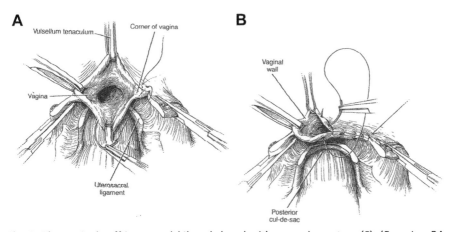

Fig. 7. The vaginal cuff is grasped (*A*) and closed with a running suture (*B*). (*From* Lee RA. Atlas of gynecologic surgery. Philadelphia: W.B. Saunders; 1992. Used with permission of Mayo Foundation for Medical Education and Research. All rights reserved.)

The pelvis is then irrigated with warm saline and all areas of dissection are inspected for hemostasis. The lap sponges are removed and counted, the self-retaining retractor is removed, and the abdominal incision is closed.

POSTOPERATIVE CARE

A Foley catheter is left in place on the day of surgery and is usually removed the following day. Traditionally, patients were maintained on intravenous fluids with nothing by mouth until they were passing flatus. However, several recent studies have shown the benefits of early feeding and ambulation and enhanced recovery protocols are available for postoperative management.[8,9] One of the key factors in postoperative management is achieving adequate pain control. Multimodal therapy is encouraged, typically with a combination of opioid narcotics and nonsteroidal anti-inflammatory agents. These can be administered intravenously immediately following the surgical procedure. Most patients are able to use oral agents within 24 to 48 hours postoperation.

COMPLICATIONS

Types of complications related to hysterectomy include infection, thromboembolism, genitourinary tract injury, gastrointestinal tract injury, nerve injury, bleeding, and cuff dehiscence. **Box 3** summarizes complication rates for abdominal hysterectomy according to a comprehensive review reported by Clarke-Pearson and Geller.[10] Infectious complications are the most common and are reported to occur in 10.5% of abdominal hysterectomy cases. Most other complications occur in the range of 1% to 2% or less. A major modifiable risk factor for complications after abdominal hysterectomy is obesity, with obese patients experiencing significantly higher rates of complications than overweight and normal weight patients.[11]

Box 3
Complications with abdominal hysterectomy

- Infectious complications
  - Cuff cellulitis: 0% to 8.3%
  - Infected pelvic hematoma/abscess: 0% to 14.6%
  - Wound infection: 0% to 22.6%
  - Urinary tract infection: 0% to 13%
  - Pneumonia: 0% to 2.2%

- Thromboembolic events: 1%

- Genitourinary tract injury
  - Bladder injury: 1% to 2%
  - Ureteral injury: 0.05% to 0.5%

- Gastrointestinal tract injury: 0.3%

- Bleeding requiring transfusion: 1% to 2%

- Nerve injury: less than 1%

- Vaginal cuff dehiscence: 0.15%

Data from Clarke-Pearson DL, Geller EJ. Complications of hysterectomy. Obstet Gynecol 2013;121:654–73.

CONTROVERSIAL ISSUES
Total Hysterectomy Versus Subtotal (Supracervical) Hysterectomy

Although often promoted with the perception of improved quality of life, sexual functioning, and pelvic support, there are no data supporting the claim of superiority of subtotal hysterectomy compared with total hysterectomy in this regard.[12] However, some patients may choose to retain the cervix and the risks and benefits of this option should be thoroughly discussed and the surgical plan individualized to meet each patient's specific needs.

Adnexal Removal

Risks and benefits of ovarian removal at the time of hysterectomy should be discussed in detail with each patient and a clear surgical plan determined before proceeding with hysterectomy. Although mortality related to ovarian cancer can be reduced with removal of the ovaries, current data suggest all-cause mortality is increased in women who have undergone ovarian removal and some women might benefit from leaving the ovaries intact at the time of hysterectomy.[13] Recent findings also suggest the potential for malignancy related to the Fallopian tube might be higher than previously thought and many women now opt for retaining the ovaries and removing the Fallopian tubes at the time of hysterectomy.[14]

SUMMARY

Hysterectomy is the most common major gynecologic procedure performed today. Although alternatives to hysterectomy have resulted in fewer procedures performed annually, and the introduction of minimally invasive techniques and continued use of vaginal hysterectomy have resulted in a lower percentage of hysterectomies being performed by the open abdominal route, pelvic disease such as large fibroids and extensive adhesive disease will require abdominal hysterectomy for treatment. Preoperative evaluation with informed consent and surgical planning are essential to properly select appropriate candidates for abdominal hysterectomy. The use of prophylactic antibiotics and thromboprophylaxis are accepted treatments to prevent postoperative complications. Attention to surgical technique is critical to prevent complications such as bleeding and injury to adjacent structures. Finally, enhanced recovery protocols should be used to provide optimal postoperative recovery for patients undergoing abdominal hysterectomy.

REFERENCES

1. Wright JD, Herzog TJ, Tsui J, et al. Nationwide trends in the performance of inpatient hysterectomy in the United States. Obstet Gynecol 2013;122:233–41.
2. Jonsdottir GM, Jorgensen S, Cohen SL, et al. Increasing minimally invasive hysterectomy: effect on cost and complications. Obstet Gynecol 2011;117:1142–9.
3. Moen M, Noone M, Cholkeri-Singh A, et al. Progressive reduction in abdominal hysterectomy rates: impact of laparoscopy, robotics and surgeon factors. J Robot Surg 2014;8:13–7.
4. Falcone T, Walters M. Hysterectomy for benign disease. Obstet Gynecol 2008;111:753–67.
5. Rahn DD, Mamik MM, Sanses TV, et al. Venous thromboembolism prophylaxis in gynecologic surgery: a systematic review. Obstet Gynecol 2011;118:1111–25.

6. Committee opinion no 610: chronic antithrombotic therapy and gynecologic surgery. Obstet Gynecol 2014;124:856–62.
7. Kumar AS, Kelleher DC, Sigle GW. Bowel preparation before elective surgery. Clin Colon Rectal Surg 2013;26:146–52.
8. Kalogera E, Bakkum-Gamez JN, Jankowski CJ, et al. Enhanced recovery in gynecologic surgery. Obstet Gynecol 2013;122:319–28.
9. Wijk L, Franzen K, Ljungqvist O, et al. Implementing a structured enhanced recovery after surgery (ERAS) protocol reduces length of stay after abdominal hysterectomy. Acta Obstet Gynecol Scand 2014;93:749–56.
10. Clarke-Pearson DL, Geller EJ. Complications of hysterectomy. Obstet Gynecol 2013;121:654–73.
11. Khavanin N, Lovecchio FC, Hanwright PJ, et al. The influence of BMI on perioperative morbidity following abdominal hysterectomy. Am J Obstet Gynecol 2013; 208:449.e1–6.
12. Lethaby A, Ivanova V, Johnson NP. Total versus subtotal hysterectomy for benign gynecological conditions. Cochrane Database Syst Rev 2006;(2):CD004993.
13. Parker WH, Feskanich D, Broder MS, et al. Long-term mortality associated with oophorectomy compared with ovarian conservation in the Nurses' Health Study. Obstet Gynecol 2013;121:709–16.
14. Salpingectomy for ovarian cancer prevention. ACOG committee opinion 620. American College of Obstetricians and Gynecologists. Obstet Gynecol 2015;(125):279–81.

Hysterectomy for Benign Conditions of the Uterus

Total Vaginal Hysterectomy

Jenifer N. Byrnes, DO, John A. Occhino, MD, MS*

KEYWORDS

- Vaginal hysterectomy • Surgical technique • Challenging situations
- Managing complications

KEY POINTS

- Vaginal hysterectomy techniques may vary slightly due to training patterns and experience but it remains the safest, most cost effective route.
- Contraindications to vaginal hysterectomy include advanced pelvic malignancy, severe endometriosis or pelvic adhesions, and adnexal disease concerning for malignancy.
- Vaginal hysterectomy can be successfully accomplished in the setting of nulliparity, enlarged uterus, obesity, and previous cesarean delivery.

HISTORICAL PERSPECTIVE

Great interest in vaginal hysterectomy has developed during the last 25 years. With broadening of indications for this operation, numerous techniques have been developed, presented, and modified, each recommended for some real or assumed advantage over those preceding it; but most have not been retained in modern gynecologic practice ... The succeeding clamp-and-ligature technique, modified by the experience of several thousand repetitions, is a rather standardized procedure offering anatomic simplicity, wide application, and great safety.
—Drs. John S. Welch and Lawrence M. Randall, Vaginal Hysterectomy at the
Mayo Clinic (1961)

The vaginal hysterectomy had humble beginnings in 1507, performed by Glacomo Berengario da Carpi for uterine prolapse.[1,2] Over the next half century, vaginal hysterectomy began being performed for additional indications, including cervical cancer, with technique modification as surgical tools were developed. The first case series documented by Senn in 1895 reported a 75% mortality rate. Cadaveric dissections, antiseptic techniques, published surgical texts and evolving surgical tools contributed to subsequent improvement in outcomes.

Division of Gynecologic Surgery, Department of Obstetrics and Gynecology, Mayo Clinic, 200 First Street Southwest, Rochester, MN 55905, USA
* Corresponding author.
E-mail address: occhino.john@mayo.edu

Obstet Gynecol Clin N Am 43 (2016) 441–462
http://dx.doi.org/10.1016/j.ogc.2016.04.004
0889-8545/16/$ – see front matter © 2016 Elsevier Inc. All rights reserved.

Abdominal hysterectomy began to gain favor in the late 1800s, but in the early twentieth century, Nobel Sproat Heaney advocated for vaginal hysterectomy for benign disease. Subsequently, Lash described a method of coring out bulky uterine tissue in 1941. In 1945, TeLinde endorsed Heaney, Danforth, and the Mayo group as expert vaginal surgeons and proponents for broader indications for vaginal hysterectomy.

TRENDS

Despite the continuous barrage of new technologies for hysterectomy, the vaginal hysterectomy remains the safest and most cost-effective approach, and is supported by numerous organizations, including the American College of Obstetricians and Gynecologists.[3] Despite this, survey data indicate only 79% of trainees feel confident performing a vaginal hysterectomy independently,[4] whereas fellowship directors believe only 20% of first year fellows were competent to perform a vaginal hysterectomy.[5] The increasing use of robotic technology has further decreased trainee exposure to vaginal hysterectomy.[6]

The number of hysterectomies performed annually in the United States continues to decline[7] and the largest proportion continue to be performed abdominally,[8] despite vaginal hysterectomy having lower complications, decreased operative time, reduced postoperative pain, and shorter hospital stay.[9–11]

High-volume surgeons are noted to have lower surgical costs, fewer complications, and better patient outcomes.[12,13] The increased use of minimally invasive laparoscopic and robotic hysterectomy has eroded the number of surgeons performing the original minimally invasive approach, vaginal hysterectomy. Surgeons, as specialists, need to reexamine previously held beliefs regarding relative contraindications to the approach. Vaginal hysterectomy can be successfully accomplished in the setting of nulliparity, enlarged uterus, obesity, and previous cesarean delivery.

Although there are data supporting vaginal hysterectomy for the treatment of early stage endometrial cancer[14] and advanced pelvic organ prolapse,[15] this article focuses on vaginal hysterectomy for benign disease.

BEST SURGICAL APPLICATIONS

Commonly accepted indications and contraindications for vaginal hysterectomy are found in **Box 1**.[3,16,17] Several studies have challenged relative contraindications to vaginal hysterectomy, including narrow pubic arch or vagina, nulliparity, history of laparotomy including cesarean delivery, absence of uterine descensus, or uterine enlargement.[10,18–24] Beyond patient factors, surgeon training and experience may affect the decision for hysterectomy route, even in patients who may be appropriate candidates for a vaginal approach.

A thorough medical and surgical history followed by a focused physical examination should be done on patients desiring hysterectomy. Particular attention should be paid to uterine size and mobility, presence of pelvic relaxation, adnexal masses, and pelvic pain during the physical examination. In an obese patient, in whom physical examination findings may be limited, preoperative imaging such as ultrasound will provide uterine dimensions and can be used to guide the choice of surgical route.[17]

TECHNIQUES
Preoperative Considerations

Screen for pregnancy
Any woman of reproductive age should be screened for pregnancy before undergoing hysterectomy and women at risk for pregnancy should be tested. Women with history

---

Box 1
Indications and contraindications for vaginal hysterectomy

Indications

- Dysfunctional uterine bleeding
- Symptomatic fibroids
- Severe dysmenorrhea
- Pelvic pain
- Uterovaginal prolapse
- Stage 1A1 cervical cancer
- Endometrial hyperplasia and early stage endometrial cancer

Contraindications

- Advanced pelvic malignancy
- Severe endometriosis or pelvic adhesions
- Adnexal disease concerning for malignancy

---

of sterilization, reliable contraceptive use, or lack of sexual activity may not require human chorionic gonadotropin (hCG) testing.

Bowel preparation
Full bowel preparation is unnecessary before simple vaginal hysterectomy. A surgeon may consider using 2 saline or tap water enemas immediately before surgery to evacuate the rectum to allow for better visualization and complete retraction of the posterior vagina.

Povidone-iodine douche
Intravaginal betadine preparation is done in the operating room before starting the procedure. Although data are lacking, some surgeons recommend betadine douche on the morning of surgery in patients without allergic contraindications to decrease microbial count.

Perineal hair removal
Hair obstructing the surgical field can be removed with the use of electric clippers, as recommended by the Centers for Disease Control and Prevention.[25]

Bladder volume
The authors prefer emptying the bladder by in-and-out catheterization before beginning the hysterectomy. Alternatively, when surgical planes are distorted, a full bladder may provide improved visualization of the bladder borders in cases of difficult dissection.

Prophylactic antibiotics
A patient undergoing hysterectomy should receive 1 dose of preoperative antibiotics according to the American College of Obstetricians and Gynecologists (ACOG) guidelines.[26]

Patient Positioning

Proper positioning is important for successful vaginal hysterectomy because it ensures adequate access to the surgical field while minimizing risk of nerve injury.[27] The patient should be placed in dorsal lithotomy position in candy-cane or yellow-fin stirrups with the buttocks at the edge of the operating table (**Fig. 1**). When using a surgical assistant, candy-cane stirrups may provide better access than yellow-fin stirrups. To decrease the risk of nerve injury, the patient's knees should be directly in line with the contralateral shoulder, with knee and hip flexion at 90° and external rotation minimized (**Fig. 2**). Evaluate for lateral leg pressure on the stirrups and add padding if necessary.

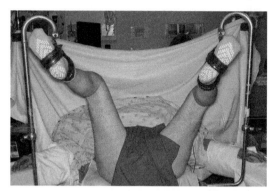

Fig. 1. Patient positioning using candy-cane stirrups. (*Used* with permission of Mayo Foundation for Medical Education and Research. All rights reserved.)

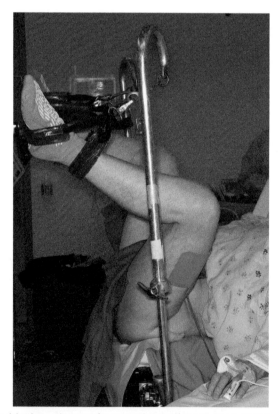

Fig. 2. Patient positioning using candy-cane stirrups (*lateral view*). (*Used* with permission of Mayo Foundation for Medical Education and Research. All rights reserved.)

Examination Under Anesthesia

Performance of a pelvic examination once the patient is under anesthesia to thoroughly evaluate the uterus and adnexa may be done, paying particular attention to access, size, and mobility. Traction on the cervix with a tenaculum can be done to help assess mobility and descent. After a thorough examination under anesthesia (EUA), some patients initially scheduled for an abdominal or laparoscopic approach may feasibly be completed vaginally. The authors routinely discuss the possibility of conversion to a vaginal hysterectomy after EUA during the office consultation and surgical consent.

Procedure Technique: Simple Vaginal Hysterectomy

Vaginal hysterectomy technique may vary slightly with training patterns and experience. Despite these minor procedural differences, it is the most minimally invasive and safest surgical approach. The following techniques reflect the authors' procedural steps.

Vaginal Incision

A weighted speculum in the posterior vagina and Deaver retractors at the 3-, 9-, and 12-o'clock positions allow for optimal visualization (**Fig. 3**). The nonperforating towel clips in **Fig. 3** are used by the authors to separate and organize the uterosacral ligament and cardinal ligament tags (see later discussion).

Grasp the cervix with 2 tenacula and palpate the cervicouterine junction (**Fig. 4**). Use firm traction while a circumferential incision is made through the vaginal mucosa sufficiently close to the distal end of the cervix to minimize risk of bladder injury (**Fig. 5**). Make the incision deep enough to reach the body of the cervix. Cut edges of the mucosa will retract superiorly under countertraction applied by Deaver retractors and the tenaculum.

Development of the Vesicovaginal Space

An assistant places traction on the cervix while the surgeon picks up the cut end of the vaginal mucosa. Mayo scissors are used to sharply dissect between the bladder and cervix (**Fig. 6**). The tip of the Mayo scissors should be directed toward the endocervical canal, away from the bladder.

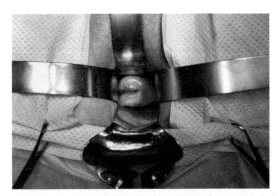

Fig. 3. Retractors placed at 3-, 9-, and 12-o'clock position for optimal visualization. (*Used with permission of Mayo Foundation for Medical Education and Research. All rights reserved.*)

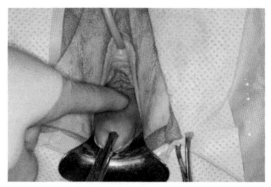

Fig. 4. Palpating the cervicouterine junction. (*Used* with permission of Mayo Foundation for Medical Education and Research. All rights reserved.)

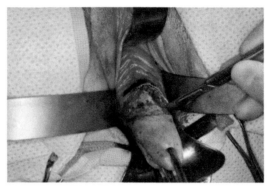

Fig. 5. Circumferential incision through anterior vaginal mucosa. (*Used* with permission of Mayo Foundation for Medical Education and Research. All rights reserved.)

Anterior Entry

An assistant places a Deaver retractor under the cut edge of the anterior vaginal wall and provides superior traction. This permits visualization of the peritoneal fold, which is grasped and incised sharply using scissors (**Fig. 7**).

Peritoneal Entry

The peritoneal opening is made sufficiently large to accommodate the Deaver retractor, which is then placed in the anterior cul-de-sac (**Fig. 8**A). Intraperitoneal location is confirmed using a right-angle Heaney retractor (**Fig. 8**B). Superior traction will elevate the base of the bladder and the ureter.

The cervix is then lifted superiorly to expose the posterior vaginal fornix. The surgeon places traction on the cut edge of the vaginal mucosa posteriorly and countertraction is applied with the cervical tenacula by the assistant. With Mayo scissors, the posterior cul-de-sac is entered (**Fig. 8**C, D).

Uterosacral Ligament

Traction is placed on the cervix toward the patient's right, and a finger is used to push the vaginal epithelium away from the cervix to expose the underlying uterosacral and cardinal ligaments (**Fig. 9**).

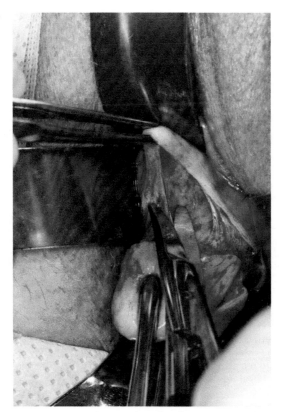

Fig. 6. Developing the vesicovaginal space. (*Used* with permission of Mayo Foundation for Medical Education and Research. All rights reserved.)

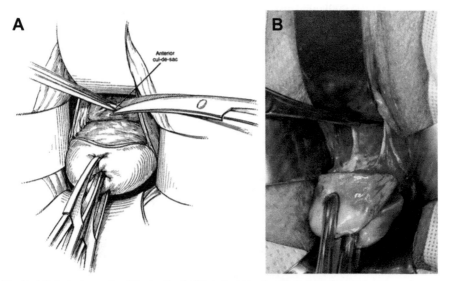

Fig. 7. (*A*) Anterior entry (illustration). (*B*) Anterior entry. ([*A*] *From* Lee RA. Atlas of gynecologic surgery. Philadelphia: W.B. Saunders; 1992. Used with permission of Mayo Foundation for Medical Education and Research. All rights reserved; and [*B*] *Used* with permission of Mayo Foundation for Medical Education and Research. All rights reserved.)

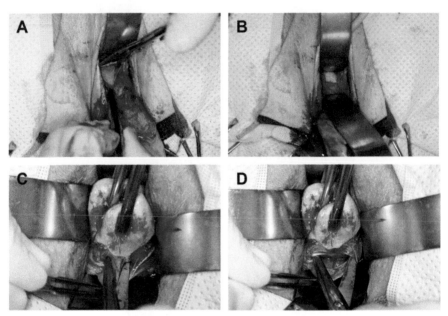

Fig. 8. (*A*) Deaver retractor in anterior cul-de-sac. (*B*) Right angle retractor used to confirm peritoneal entry. (*C*) Posterior entry: incise vaginal mucosa. (*D*) Posterior entry: enlarge incision to accommodate retractor. (*Used* with permission of Mayo Foundation for Medical Education and Research. All rights reserved.)

A Heaney clamp is placed on the left uterosacral ligament close to the vaginal epithelium, with the curved tip directed superiorly (**Fig. 10**). The ligament is divided and the incision is continued around the tip of the forceps to accommodate the placement of a tie with a short pedicle.

A ligature using polyglactin 910 (No. 0) suture is passed through the tissues behind the Heaney clamp in the middle of the ligament and tied once. Then 1 end of the suture is carried around the superior end of the pedicle and tied with 3 additional secure knots. As the first of these is tied, the Heaney clamp is slowly opened to permit tightening of the tissues while preventing retraction of the vessels

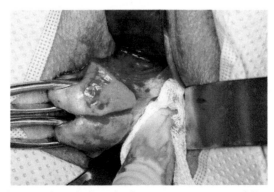

Fig. 9. Gently push vaginal epithelium back to expose uterosacral ligaments. (*Used* with permission of Mayo Foundation for Medical Education and Research. All rights reserved.)

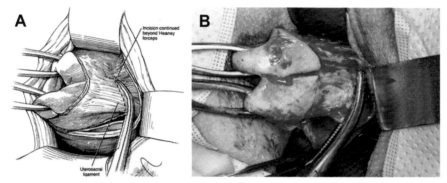

Fig. 10. (*A*) Clamping the uterosacral ligament (illustration). (*B*) Clamping the uterosacral ligament. ([*A*] *From* Lee RA. Atlas of gynecologic surgery. Philadelphia: W.B. Saunders; 1992. Used with permission of Mayo Foundation for Medical Education and Research. All rights reserved; and [*B*] *Used* with permission of Mayo Foundation for Medical Education and Research. All rights reserved.)

before the suture is secured (**Fig. 11**). For all pedicle ligation, the authors use this modified Heaney ligature technique; however, any secure ligature will suffice.

Once tied, the end of the suture is left long and tagged for later identification during suspension of the vaginal cuff. The tagged end of the suture is tucked behind the weighted speculum. The authors use straight clamps to identify the uterosacral ligaments and curved clamps to identify the cardinal-vascular pedicles.

Ureteral Identification or Palpation

Palpate the left ureter by inserting the left index finger through the anterior cul-de-sac beneath the Deaver retractor, elevating the bladder, and palpating the lower segment of the left ureter between the index finger and the surface of the Deaver retractor in the 3-o'clock position (**Fig. 12**) A characteristic pop can be heard when the ureter is snapped between the index finger and the retractor.

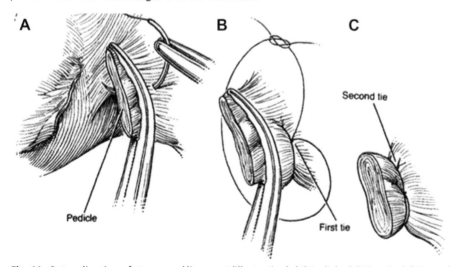

Fig. 11. Suture ligation of uterosacral ligament (illustration). (*A*) Pedicle. (*B*) First tie. (*C*) Second tie. (*From* Lee RA. Atlas of gynecologic surgery. Philadelphia: W.B. Saunders; 1992. Used with permission of Mayo Foundation for Medical Education and Research. All rights reserved.)

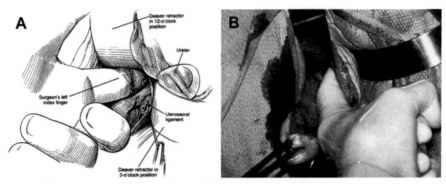

Fig. 12. (*A*) Palpating the ureter (illustration). (*B*) Palpating the ureter. ([*A*] *From* Lee RA. Atlas of gynecologic surgery. Philadelphia: W.B. Saunders; 1992. Used with permission of Mayo Foundation for Medical Education and Research. All rights reserved; and [*B*] *Used* with permission of Mayo Foundation for Medical Education and Research. All rights reserved.)

Cardinal Ligament

Once ureteral location is known, place the Heaney clamp on the lower portion of the cardinal ligament (**Fig. 13**), with the clamp pointed toward the endocervical canal, directed away from the ureter. Incise and suture-ligate the cardinal ligament, tagging the suture in a similar fashion as with the uterosacral ligament, and letting it hang over the towel clamp placed on the drape.

The last clamp on the cardinal ligament brings together the peritoneum of the anterior and posterior cul-de-sacs (**Fig. 14**). The uterine artery is typically located in this pedicle.

This pedicle is cut and suture-ligated, and the distal ends of the tie are included in the curved clamp (the 2 pedicles represent the cardinal ligament).

The procedure described previously is then repeated on the patient's right side, including palpation of the ureter. Of note, the streamlined technique used by the authors allows for an efficient hysterectomy because all connective tissue is ligated and divided 1 side at a time.

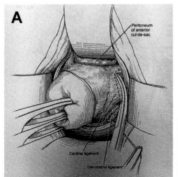
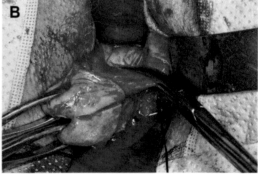

Fig. 13. (*A*) Clamping the lower portion of cardinal ligament (illustration). (*B*) Clamping the lower portion of cardinal ligament. ([*A*] *From* Lee RA. Atlas of gynecologic surgery. Philadelphia: W.B. Saunders; 1992. Used with permission of Mayo Foundation for Medical Education and Research. All rights reserved; and [*B*] *Used* with permission of Mayo Foundation for Medical Education and Research. All rights reserved.)

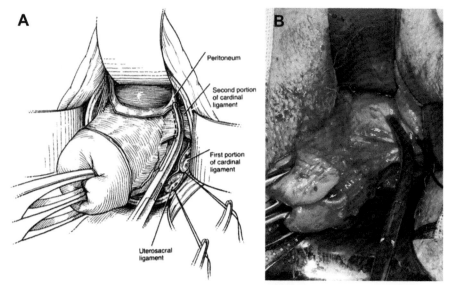

Fig. 14. (*A*) Clamping the upper portion of cardinal ligament (illustration). (*B*) Clamping the upper portion of cardinal ligament. ([*A*] *From* Lee RA. Atlas of gynecologic surgery. Philadelphia: W.B. Saunders; 1992. Used with permission of Mayo Foundation for Medical Education and Research. All rights reserved; and [*B*] *Used* with permission of Mayo Foundation for Medical Education and Research. All rights reserved.)

Utero-Ovarian Pedicle

At this point, the uterus is held in place by the remaining portions of the broad ligament inferior to the round ligament and utero-ovarian ligament. Uterine mobility should allow delivery of the uterine fundus to deliver the through the posterior cul-de-sac into the vagina.

The surgeon's left hand is placed behind the uterus and the Heaney clamp is inserted from above, clamping the right utero-ovarian pedicle. The surgeon's fingers are used to prevent inadvertent injury to adjacent bowel (**Fig. 15**). This clamp includes the fallopian tube, round ligament, and any remaining portion of the broad ligament. This procedure is repeated on the left utero-ovarian pedicle.

Evaluate for Hemostasis

The uterus is removed and sent for pathologic evaluation. All pedicles are inspected for hemostasis. If necessary, placement of interrupted absorbable sutures may be used until hemostasis is achieved. Frequently, bleeding is noted along the posterior vaginal cuff, and electrocautery is used for obtaining hemostasis. At this point, a vaginal pack is used to help elevate the bowel away from the operative field.

Addressing the Adnexa

In most cases, removal of adnexal structures can be successfully accomplished transvaginally.[28] It is the authors' practice to perform prophylactic salpingectomy for ovarian cancer prevention at the time of hysterectomy, as recommended by ACOG.[29] We use Heaney clamps and suture ligature whenever possible (**Fig. 16**). Alternatively, electrocautery, vessel sealing devices,[30] or Endoloop suture ligatures can be used.

If the patient requires salpingo-oophorectomy, the utero-ovarian pedicle is grasped with an Allis clamp, and gentle traction is placed on the adnexa. Russian forceps are

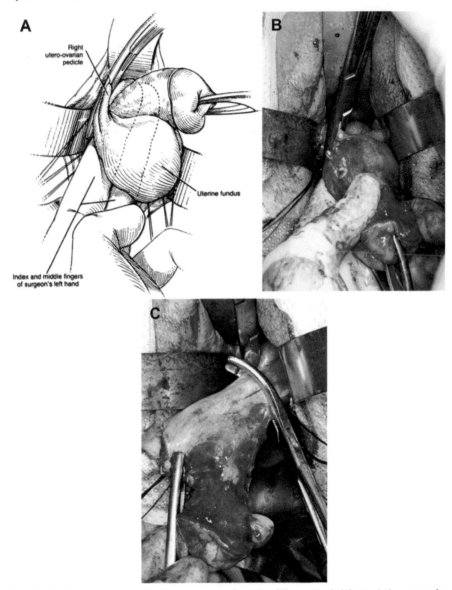

Fig. 15. (*A*) Hand placement for utero-ovarian clamping (illustration). (*B*) Hand placement for utero-ovarian clamping. (*C*) Clamp placement on utero-ovarian ligament. ([*A*] *From* Lee RA. Atlas of gynecologic surgery. Philadelphia: W.B. Saunders; 1992. Used with permission of Mayo Foundation for Medical Education and Research. All rights reserved; and [*B, C*] *Used* with permission of Mayo Foundation for Medical Education and Research. All rights reserved.)

used to grasp the fallopian tube, which routinely lies atop the ovary. The tube and ovary are grasped with an additional Allis clamp. This Allis is used to pull the adnexa toward the midline, exposing the infundibulopelvic ligament containing the ovarian vessels. A Heaney clamp is placed across the infundibulopelvic ligament (**Fig. 17**), paying special attention to avoid the ureter. After resection, the pedicle is doubly ligated, initially using a heavy, absorbable free tie, followed by suture-ligation. The contralateral tube and ovary can be removed in a similar fashion.

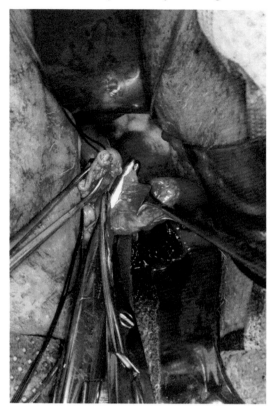

Fig. 16. Clamp placement for salpingectomy. (*Used* with permission of Mayo Foundation for Medical Education and Research. All rights reserved.)

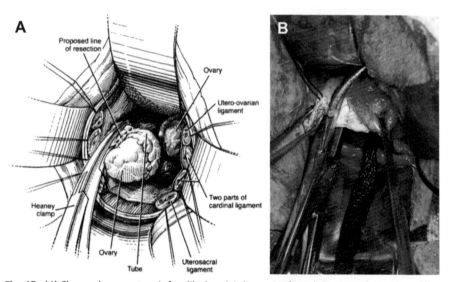

Fig. 17. (*A*) Clamp placement on infundibulopelvic ligament for salpingo-oophorectomy (illustration). (*B*) Clamp placement on infundibulopelvic ligament for salpingo-oophorectomy. ([*A*] *From* Lee RA. Atlas of gynecologic surgery. Philadelphia: W.B. Saunders; 1992. Used with permission of Mayo Foundation for Medical Education and Research. All rights reserved; and [*B*] *Used* with permission of Mayo Foundation for Medical Education and Research. All rights reserved.)

Modified McCall Apical Suspension

At the time of all vaginal hysterectomies, including those without significant amounts of pelvic organ prolapse, the authors prophylactically resuspend the vaginal cuff using a modified-McCall technique (**Fig. 18**). This uses the uterosacral ligaments for suspension and closes the enterocele space. A heavy polyglactin 910 suture (No. 1) is placed through the posterior vaginal cuff at the midline, and exits intraperitoneally (**Fig. 19**). An assistant gives traction on the previously tagged left uterosacral ligament and an intraperitoneal bite of the ligament is taken (**Fig. 20**). The same suture is used to reef across the peritoneum of the rectum, toward the patient's right side (**Fig. 21**). Traction is given on the right uterosacral ligament (previously tagged) and a bite of this is taken (**Fig. 22**). Still using the same suture, bring it back through the posterior vaginal cuff, adjacent to where it initially entered (**Fig. 23**). This is tagged and will be tied later. The authors routinely place a second suture in a similar fashion for additional support.

Reperitonealization

Closure of the peritoneum is done in a purse-string fashion, incorporating a portion of the uterosacral ligaments cephalad to the previously placed modified-McCall sutures. The tail of suture is left long to allow it to be brought through the vaginal cuff after the peritoneum is closed. The vaginal pack is now removed and the peritoneal closure suture is tied. The end with the needle is brought through the vaginal cuff, while a bare needle is used to bring the tail end through the vaginal cuff, adjacent to it.

The reperitonealization and modified-McCall sutures are tied and cystoscopy is performed for evaluation of ureteral function. The authors routinely use cystoscopy at the time of vaginal hysterectomy, particularly following modified-McCall culdosuspension and on completion of the procedure.

Vaginal Cuff Closure

Again, hemostasis is evaluated and managed using electrocautery or suture placement. Close the vaginal cuff with interrupted absorbable sutures (No. 1) starting at

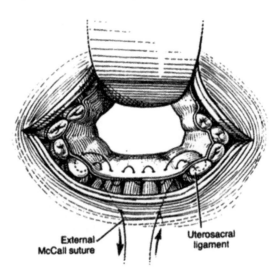

Fig. 18. McCall culdoplasty (illustration). (*From* Lee RA. Atlas of gynecologic surgery. Philadelphia: W.B. Saunders; 1992. Used with permission of Mayo Foundation for Medical Education and Research. All rights reserved.)

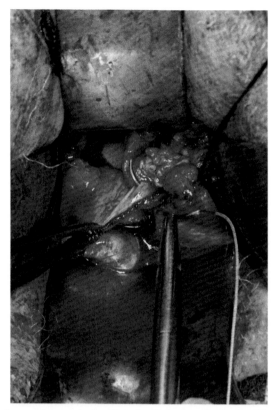

Fig. 19. Step 1: Suture enters vaginal cuff and exits intraperitoneally. (*Used* with permission of Mayo Foundation for Medical Education and Research. All rights reserved.)

the patient's left cuff angle. Place a suture through the posterior vaginal wall. With traction on the uterosacral ligament, a distal bite of the ligament is obtained for additional support, followed by a bite of the tagged cardinal ligament. Finally, it is brought through the anterior vaginal wall and tied. Placement of 2 additional interrupted sutures is done to close the cuff on the patient's left side. The right side of the vaginal vault is closed in a similar fashion, incorporating the uterosacral and cardinal ligaments into the cuff closure.

Summary and Key Points

Most patients requiring hysterectomy for benign disease are candidates for a vaginal approach. Using the systematic techniques discussed can ensure a safe, easy procedure in most cases. The next section discusses ways to optimize vaginal hysterectomy utilization in challenging situations.

CHALLENGING SITUATIONS
Previous Pelvic Surgery or Cesarean Delivery

Careful dissection and knowledge of surgical planes are essential to avoid incidental cystotomy. Distending the bladder by back-filling the Foley catheter may assist in identifying bladder anatomy in uncertain cases. If scarring is preventing successful anterior entry, the posterior cul-de-sac can be entered and ligation of the uterosacral ligaments bilaterally can be done to facilitate mobility and visualization.

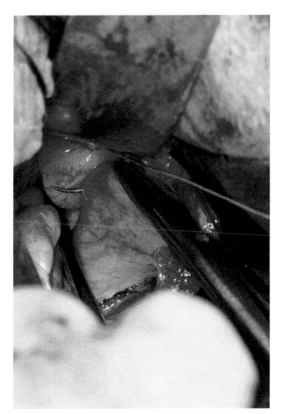

Fig. 20. Step 2: Intraperitoneal bite of uterosacral ligament. (*Used* with permission of Mayo Foundation for Medical Education and Research. All rights reserved.)

Cervical Elongation

The presence of cervical elongation may not be known before surgery and patience is the key to a successful vaginal hysterectomy in these cases. Continue the procedure in a stepwise fashion, keeping in mind that the anterior and posterior peritoneal entry will occur much higher than usual. The cervix and/or uterus may be bivalved to improve access to the peritoneal reflection once the uterine arteries have been ligated bilaterally.

Enlarged Uterus

Patients with enlarged uteri should be counseled on options to aid in successful minimally invasive hysterectomy. Morcellation, the division of tissue into smaller fragments, is a volume reduction technique.[10] In 2014, the US Food and Drug Administration (FDA) released a statement on safety concerns with power morcellation techniques due to risk of disseminated leiomyosarcoma.[31,32] Although vaginal hysterectomy does not use power morcellators, it is important to discuss volume reduction techniques with patients before surgery when feasible.

Bimanual EUA should be used to estimate uterine size. Vaginal hysterectomy can be performed successfully in uteri up to 16 to 18 weeks in size with the use of morcellation techniques, provided access to the cardinal and uterosacral ligaments can be achieved. This should not be considered in cases with suspected uterine malignancy.

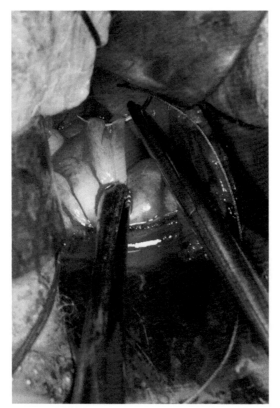

Fig. 21. Step 3: Reef across posterior peritoneum. (*Used* with permission of Mayo Foundation for Medical Education and Research. All rights reserved.)

Place tenacula on each side of the cervix and apply lateral traction while vertically incising the cervix up to the cervicouterine junction. Sharp debulking of the uterus using a scalpel can be done by removing any visible uterine fibroids as they are encountered. This is done until the uterus can be delivered through the vaginal opening. Careful attention must be paid to avoiding bowel injury while using this technique.

Alternatively, intramyometrial coring as described by Kovac[33] can be used. In this technique, the central bulk of the myometrium is excised, leaving a more readily flexible uterine shell.

Obese Body Habitus

Obesity is associated with an increased risk of perioperative complications, including infectious morbidity.[17] Vaginal surgery can be challenging in obese women because soft tissue can impair visualization. Adequate exposure is essential and retractor size and type should be modified as needed to complete the surgery safely. This may include the use of a self-retaining retractor or additional assistance in the operative suite. Using surgical drapes to secure the weighted vaginal speculum (**Fig. 24**) can also be helpful, both in cases of obesity and in advanced posterior wall prolapse. An assistant familiar with anatomy and the surgical procedure may also make these technically challenging cases more feasible.

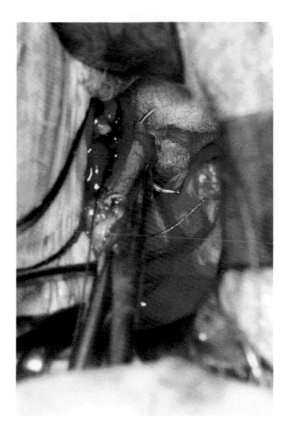

Fig. 22. Step 4: Intraperitoneal bite of contralateral uterosacral ligament. (*Used* with permission of Mayo Foundation for Medical Education and Research. All rights reserved.)

COMPLICATIONS
Bladder Injury

Incidental cystotomy is reported to occur in 1.2% to 4% of vaginal hysterectomies.[34] Intraoperative identification of injury is essential to help decrease the risk of vesicovaginal fistula formation. The authors routinely perform cystoscopy at the time of hysterectomy, which has been shown to increase the intraoperative detection rate of urinary tract injuries.[35] If bladder injury is suspected, a Foley catheter can be used to back-fill the bladder with approximately 300 cc of fluid, typically stained with methylene blue, to evaluate for extravasation. If a cystotomy is identified, it is best to tag the location with a suture and proceed with hysterectomy completion. Removal of the uterus facilitates visualization and allows any additional bladder injuries to be repaired at the same time.

The cystotomy is identified by locating the previously placed suture tag. The edges are identified and the cystotomy is closed in a 2-layer fashion. The first layer is closed with an absorbable suture (usually 2–0 or 3–0), in a running fashion that incorporates bladder epithelium. This is followed by an imbricating layer of running absorbable suture. When possible, the authors mobilize the anterior bladder peritoneum and secure this over the cystotomy closure as an additional barrier to fistula formation. Cystoscopy should be performed after cystotomy repair to evaluate for a watertight

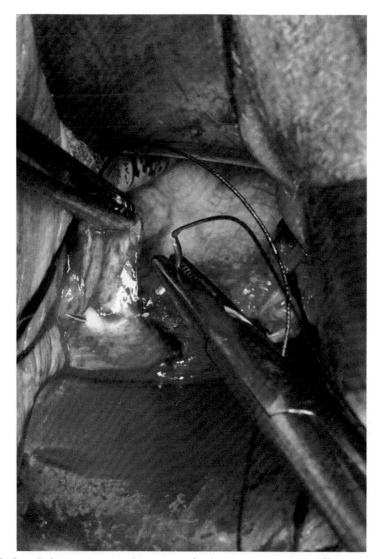

Fig. 23. Step 5: Suture enters peritoneum and exits posterior vaginal cuff on contralateral side. (*Used* with permission of Mayo Foundation for Medical Education and Research. All rights reserved.)

seal and ensure bilateral ureteral function. Prolonged bladder draining should follow for 5 to 10 days using a transurethral catheter.

Ureteral Injury

Ureteral injury is less common than cystotomy, and is estimated at 0.05% to 0.5%.[34] Ureteral injuries can occur as a result of ligation, transection, crush injury, suture entrapment, or thermal damage. During hysterectomy, this is most likely to occur during uterine artery or infundibulopelvic ligament ligation or during suspension of the vaginal cuff to the uterosacral ligaments. Rates of injury due to suture entrapment

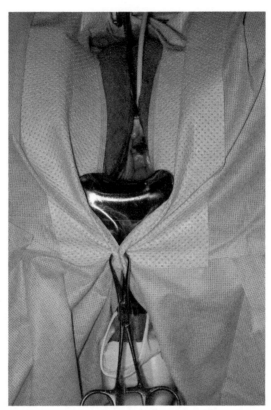

Fig. 24. Securing weighted speculum with drapes. (*Used* with permission of Mayo Foundation for Medical Education and Research. All rights reserved.)

from uterosacral ligament suspension are reported to be as high as 11%.[36] Intraoperative cystoscopy has a sensitivity of 94.4% and specificity of 99.5% in detecting ureteral obstruction, and provides an opportunity for early intervention.[37]

The authors use cystoscopy liberally because most ureteral injuries occur in women without risk factors. If cystoscopy is not routinely done, it should be performed if ureteral injury is suspected. Previously, intravenous administration of indigo carmine was used to aid ureteral efflux visualization. In 2014, the FDA announced a shortage of indigo carmine, prompting the use of alterative medications. One alternative is a 10% preparation of sodium fluorescein (0.25 to 1 mL administered intravenously), which will stain the ureteral jets a brilliant yellow minutes after injection.[38] The authors prefer phenazopyridine 100 mg by mouth approximately 30 to 60 minutes before surgery.

SUMMARY

As minimally invasive technology continues to be developed and refined, surgeons must be discerning in choosing the safest, cost-effective surgical approach associated with the best outcomes for each individual patient. Vaginal hysterectomy can be successfully accomplished even in challenging situations, such as previous pelvic surgery, nulliparity, uterine enlargement, or obesity. Vaginal hysterectomy should be considered the primary route for treatment of benign disease.

REFERENCES

1. Sparić R, Hudelist G, Berisava M, et al. Hysterectomy throughout history. Acta Chir Iugosl 2011;58(4):9–14.
2. Tizzano AP, Walters MD. Hysterectomy for benign disease. Philadelphia: Saunders, an imprint of Elsevier Inc; 2010.
3. ACOG Committee Opinion No. 444: choosing the route of hysterectomy for benign disease. Obstet Gynecol 2009;114(5):1156–8.
4. Kenton K, Sultana C, Rogers RG, et al, American Urogynecologic Society EducationCommittee. How well are we training residents in female pelvic medicine and reconstructive surgery? Am J Obstet Gynecol 2008;198(5): 567.e1–4.
5. Guntupalli SR, Doo DW, Guy M, et al. Preparedness of Obstetrics and Gynecology Residents for Fellowship Training. Obstet Gynecol 2015;126(3):559–68.
6. Jeppson PC, Rahimi S, Gattoc L, et al. Impact of robotic technology on hysterectomy route and associated implications for resident education. Am J Obstet Gynecol 2015;212(2):196.e1–6.
7. Merrill RM. Hysterectomy surveillance in the United States, 1997 through 2005. Med Sci Monit 2008;14(1):CR24–31.
8. Wu JM, Wechter ME, Geller EJ, et al. Hysterectomy rates in the United States, 2003. Obstet Gynecol 2007;110(5):1091–5.
9. Sesti F, Calonzi F, Ruggeri V, et al. A comparison of vaginal, laparoscopic-assisted vaginal, and minilaparotomy hysterectomies for enlarged myomatous uteri. Int J Gynaecol Obstet 2008;103(3):227–31.
10. Benassi L, Rossi T, Kaihura CT, et al. Abdominal or vaginal hysterectomy for enlarged uteri: a randomized clinical trial. Am J Obstet Gynecol 2002;187(6): 1561–5.
11. Schindlbeck C, Klauser K, Dian D, et al. Comparison of total laparoscopic, vaginal and abdominal hysterectomy. Arch Gynecol Obstet 2008;277(4):331–7.
12. Rogo-Gupta LJ, Lewin SN, Kim JH, et al. The effect of surgeon volume on outcomes and resource use for vaginal hysterectomy. Obstet Gynecol 2010; 116(6):1341–7.
13. Boyd LR, Novetsky AP, Curtin JP. Effect of surgical volume on route of hysterectomy and short-term morbidity. Obstet Gynecol 2010;116(4):909–15.
14. Zanagnolo V, Magrina JF. Carcinoma of the endometrium treated only by vaginal route. Best Pract Res Clin Obstet Gynaecol 2011;25(2):239–45.
15. Jeppson PC, Sung VW. Hysterectomy for pelvic organ prolapse: indications and techniques. Clin Obstet Gynecol 2014;57(1):72–82.
16. Webb MJ, Cliby WA, Gostout BS, et al. Mayo Clinic manual of pelvic surgery. 2nd edition. Philadelphia: Lippincott Williams & Wilkins; 2000.
17. Committee on Gynecologic Practice. Committee opinion no. 619: Gynecologic surgery in the obese woman. Obstet Gynecol 2015;125(1):274–8.
18. Rooney CM, Crawford AT, Vassallo BJ, et al. Is previous cesarean section a risk for incidental cystotomy at the time of hysterectomy? A case-controlled study. Am J Obstet Gynecol 2005;193(6):2041–4.
19. Figueiredo O, Figueiredo EG, Figueiredo PG, et al. Vaginal removal of the benign nonprolapsed uterus: experience with 300 consecutive operations. Obstet Gynecol 1999;94(3):348–51.
20. Doucette RC, Sharp HT, Alder SC. Challenging generally accepted contraindications to vaginal hysterectomy. Am J Obstet Gynecol 2001;184(7): 1386–9 [discussion: 90–1].

21. Paparella P, Sizzi O, Rossetti A, et al. Vaginal hysterectomy in generally consid-ered contraindications to vaginal surgery. Arch Gynecol Obstet 2004;270(2): 104–9.
22. Tohic AL, Dhainaut C, Yazbeck C, et al. Hysterectomy for benign uterine pathology among women without previous vaginal delivery. Obstet Gynecol 2008;111(4):829–37.
23. Unger JB, Meeks GR. Vaginal hysterectomy in women with history of previous cesarean delivery. Am J Obstet Gynecol 1998;179(6 Pt 1):1473–8.
24. Unger JB. Vaginal hysterectomy for the woman with a moderately enlarged uterus weighing 200 to 700 grams. Am J Obstet Gynecol 1999;180(6 Pt 1):1337–44.
25. Reichman DE, Greenberg JA. Reducing surgical site infections: a review. Rev Obstet Gynecol 2009;2(4):212–21.
26. ACOG Committee on Practice Bulletins–Gynecology. ACOG practice bulletin No. 104: antibiotic prophylaxis for gynecologic procedures. Obstet Gynecol 2009; 113(5):1180–9.
27. Kim-Fine S, Occhino JA, Gebhart JB. Difficult vaginal hysterectomy. Expert Rev Obstet Gynecol 2013;8(4):369–77.
28. Camanni M, Mistrangelo E, Febo G, et al. Prophylactic bilateral oophorectomy during vaginal hysterectomy for benign pathology. Arch Gynecol Obstet 2009; 280(1):87–90.
29. Committee on Gynecologic Practice. Committee opinion no. 620: Salpingectomy for ovarian cancer prevention. Obstet Gynecol 2015;125(1):279–81.
30. Kroft J, Selk A. Energy-based vessel sealing in vaginal hysterectomy: a system-atic review and meta-analysis. Obstet Gynecol 2011;118(5):1127–36.
31. Desai VB, Guo XM, Xu X. Alterations in surgical technique after FDA statement on power morcellation. Am J Obstet Gynecol 2015;212(5):685–7.
32. Ton R, Kilic GS, Phelps JY. A medical-legal review of power morcellation in the face of the recent FDA warning and litigation. J Minim Invasive Gynecol 2015; 22(4):564–72.
33. Kovac SR. Intramyometrial coring as an adjunct to vaginal hysterectomy. Obstet Gynecol 1986;67(1):131–6.
34. Clarke-Pearson DL, Geller EJ. Complications of hysterectomy. Obstet Gynecol 2013;121(3):654–73.
35. Teeluckdharry B, Gilmour D, Flowerdew G. Urinary Tract Injury at Benign Gynecologic Surgery and the Role of Cystoscopy: A Systematic Review and Meta-analysis. Obstet Gynecol 2015;126(6):1161–9.
36. Walters MD, Ridgeway BM. Surgical treatment of vaginal apex prolapse. Obstet Gynecol 2013;121(2 Pt 1):354–74.
37. Gustilo-Ashby AM, Jelovsek JE, Barber MD, et al. The incidence of ureteral obstruction and the value of intraoperative cystoscopy during vaginal surgery for pelvic organ prolapse. Am J Obstet Gynecol 2006;194(5):1478–85.
38. Doyle PJ, Lipetskaia L, Duecy E, et al. Sodium fluorescein use during intraoper-ative cystoscopy. Obstet Gynecol 2015;125(3):548–50.

Total Laparoscopic Hysterectomy and Laparoscopic-Assisted Vaginal Hysterectomy

Cara R. King, DO, MS, Dobie Giles, MD, MS*

KEYWORDS

- Laparoscopic hysterectomy • Laparoscopic assisted vaginal hysterectomy
- Minimally invasive surgery • Vaginal surgery • Laparoscopy

KEY POINTS

- When vaginal hysterectomy is not possible, laparoscopic hysterectomy and laparoscopic-assisted vaginal hysterectomy are excellent methods for removal of the uterus.
- Poor descent of the uterus, as with fibroids, or need to evaluate the pelvis, as with endometriosis, are examples of indications for a laparoscopic approach.
- Advanced laparoscopic skills are often required to complete a total laparoscopic hysterectomy. Completion of the hysterectomy vaginally is an option, with the amount of vaginal dissection required dependent on the laparoscopic portion.
- Attention to sound surgical steps, including visualization, traction, and hemostasis, is the key to success. Cystoscopy is recommended at case completion.
- Patients with a successful minimally invasive approach will return to work sooner with decreased pain and a shorter hospital stay when compared with those who undergo abdominal hysterectomy.

HISTORICAL PERSPECTIVE

Hysterectomies have been reported as early as 50 BC by Themison and 120 AD by Soranus, but it was not until 1813 that Conrad Langenbeck performed the first planned vaginal hysterectomy in modern times.[1,2] Charles Clay is credited with performing the first abdominal hysterectomy in Manchester, England in 1839.[1] Thomas Keith started to incorporate aseptic techniques with the procedure and by 1910 had decreased the mortality of vaginal hysterectomy down to 2.5%.[2] Despite improvements in vaginal

Division of Gynecology and Gynecologic Subspecialties, Department of Obstetrics and Gynecology, University of Wisconsin-Madison, 600 Highland Avenue, CSC H4/630, Madison, WI 53792, USA
* Corresponding author.
E-mail address: Giles2@wisc.edu

Obstet Gynecol Clin N Am 43 (2016) 463–478
http://dx.doi.org/10.1016/j.ogc.2016.04.005
0889-8545/16/$ – see front matter © 2016 Elsevier Inc. All rights reserved.

obgyn.theclinics.com

surgery over time, the open abdominal approach to hysterectomies accounted for 75% of the cases for removal of the uterus.[2]

Gynecologists were the pioneers in laparoscopy; as technology advanced, so did the surgical techniques. Harry Reich performed the first laparoscopic hysterectomy in 1989.[1,3] In less than a year, Kovac and colleagues[4] reported the first laparoscopic-assisted vaginal hysterectomy. As more surgeons incorporated laparoscopic techniques into their hysterectomies, a classification system was developed to provide consistency in terminology (**Table 1**).[5] The use of the laparoscope allowed for removal of the uterus in cases whereby it could not be completed solely through the vagina or in cases whereby evaluation of the pelvic structures was necessary.

Table 1	
Classification system for laparoscopically directed and assisted total hysterectomy	
Type 0	Laparoscopically directed preparation for vaginal hysterectomy
Type I[a]	Dissection up to but not including uterine arteries
Type IA	Ovarian artery pedicles only
Type IB[b]	A + anterior structures
Type IC	A + posterior culdotomy
Type ID[b]	A + anterior structures and posterior culdotomy
Type II[a]	Type I + uterine artery and vein occlusion, unilateral or bilateral
Type IIA	Ovarian artery pedicles plus unilateral or bilateral uterine artery and vein occlusion only
Type IIB[b]	A + anterior structures
Type IIC	A + posterior culdotomy
Type ID[b]	A + anterior structures and posterior culdotomy
Type III[a]	Type II + portion of cardinal-uterosacral ligament complex; unilateral or bilateral, plus
Type IIIA	Uterine and ovarian artery pedicles with unilateral or bilateral portion of the cardinal-uterosacral complex only
Type IIIB[b]	A + anterior structures
Type IIIC	A + posterior culdotomy
Type IIID[b]	A + anterior structures and posterior culdotomy
Type IV[a]	Type III + total cardinal-uterosacral ligament complex; unilateral or bilateral, plus
Type IVA	Uterine and ovarian artery pedicles with unilateral or bilateral detachment of the total cardinal-uterosacral ligament complex only
Type IVB[b]	A + anterior structures
Type IVC	A + posterior culdotomy
Type IVD[b]	A + anterior structures and posterior culdotomy
Type IVE	Laparoscopically directed removal of entire uterus

The system describes the portion of the procedure completed laparoscopically.

[a] A suffix o may be added if unilateral or bilateral oophorectomy is performed concomitantly (eg, type IoA).

[b] The B and D subgroups may be further subclassified according to the degree of dissection involving the bladder and whether an anterior culdotomy is created: (1) incision of vesicouterine peritoneum only, (2) dissection of any portion of bladder from cervix, (3) creation of an anterior culdotomy.

From Munro MG, Parker WH. A classification system for laparoscopic hysterectomy. Obstet Gynecol 1993;82(4 Pt 1):625; with permission.

INDICATIONS/CONTRAINDICATIONS

The most common indications for hysterectomy include leiomyoma, abnormal vaginal bleeding, endometriosis, adenomyosis, pelvic organ prolapse, and gynecologic cancer.[6] A laparoscopic approach may provide an advantage in women with extrauterine pelvic pathology (endometriosis, significant adhesive disease) or chronic pelvic pain. A large uterine size may also be an indication for a laparoscopic approach; however, the upper limit is dictated by a multitude of factors, including skill of the surgeon, location of uterine bulk, uterine descent, and access to uterine vasculature.[7]

There are few contraindications to a laparoscopic approach in the hands of a skilled laparoscopic surgeon (**Table 2**). The primary limiting factor predicting a successful minimally invasive approach remains the experience and skill level of the surgeon. Medical conditions that preclude laparoscopy include severe cardiopulmonary pathologies with intolerance to increased intra-abdominal pressure or Trendelenburg positioning, which may limit visualization.[8] Laparoscopic hysterectomy should also be approached with caution in women with suspected uterine or adnexal malignancy that cannot be removed intact. Tissue extraction should always be thoughtful and well planned. When tissue fractionation is contraindicated and vaginal retrieval is not successful, consideration should be made for mini-laparotomy or laparotomy.

TRENDS

According to the Nationwide Inpatient Sample, the number of inpatient hysterectomies performed in the United States peaked in 2002 with 681,234 and declined to 433,621 in 2010.[6] Vaginal hysterectomy has declined from 24.8% in 1998 to 16.7% in 2010.[6] There was a peak in laparoscopic hysterectomy in 2006 at 15.5%, but this has declined to 8.6% in 2010.[6] Part of this decline can be accounted for in the increase in robotic hysterectomy from 0.9% in 2008% to 8.2% in 2010.[6] These numbers do not account for the increasing number of patients discharged home the same day of surgery (same-day hysterectomy). In addition, there are more options for uterine-sparing management that may decrease the total number of hysterectomies performed, such as endometrial ablation, uterine artery embolization, and medical therapy.

TECHNIQUE/PROCEDURE
Preparation

A thorough and meticulous presurgical evaluation is pivotal for a successful operative and postoperative course. Many complications can be minimized or eliminated with a strategic preoperative workup and surgical planning. Aside from the obvious history regarding indications for hysterectomy, details should also be obtained regarding additional comorbidities and associated medications, personal or family history for thromboembolism, and personal or family history of anesthesia-related complications.

Table 2
Indications and contraindications to laparoscopic approach to hysterectomy

Indications	Contraindications
Extrauterine pelvic pathology	Inadequate surgical skill
Significant adhesive disease	Significant cardiopulmonary disease
Large uterine size	Suspicious or known gynecologic malignancy and inability to remove specimen intact

Women with significant comorbidities should be referred for the appropriate consultations for surgical optimization. Correction of anemia, uncontrolled diabetes, and hypertension is ideal before elective hysterectomies are performed. An in-depth surgical history should also be obtained, and all previous abdominal operative reports should be reviewed. Details of previous surgical findings offer great insight on the anticipated surgical complexity of future procedures. If significant bowel or bladder adhesions are suspected, appropriate surgical backup from colorectal surgery or urology should be arranged pending your surgical skill level and comfort.

When physical examination is limited by body habitus or intolerance of the examination, additional imaging with an ultrasound or MRI is often helpful. When fibroids are present and tissue fractionation is anticipated, the authors' facility also requires a preoperative endometrial biopsy regardless of bleeding profile.

Routine mechanical bowel preparation (MBP) is no longer standard practice before routine laparoscopic hysterectomy. The use of preoperative MBP provides theoretic advantages, including ease of bowel manipulation, increased pelvic visualization, and reduction in postoperative infection outcomes if bowel injury occurs; however, current literature has not shown an improvement in surgical or postoperative outcomes.[9–12] Despite the current evidence, some experts think there is benefit in the use of MBP in advanced laparoscopic surgery whereby concern for bowel involvement is palpated on examination (rectal nodule, uterosacral tethering, obliterated cul-de-sac) or through preoperative imaging.

Table 3 shows a list of standard equipment for a total laparoscopic hysterectomy.

Patient Positioning

Methodical patient positioning should be executed before every case to provide optimal patient safety and enhanced surgeon visualization and access to the field (**Fig. 1**). Patients should be placed on a foam pad or its equivalent to minimize slippage while in Trendelenburg position. Sequential compression devices are routinely placed and activated on entry into the operating room. Following induction of general anesthesia and successful intubation, an orogastric tube is placed to allow adequate

Table 3
Standard equipment for total laparoscopic hysterectomy

Standard Equipment	Comments
Uterine manipulator	RUMI (Cooper Surgical, Trumbull, CT)
Catheter	14F or 16F Foley
0° and 30° laparoscope	10-mm and 5-mm Laparoscopes available in room; 10 mm 0° most commonly used
One 12-mm trocar, three 5-mm trocars	Prefer open Hasson entry
2 Atraumatic graspers	—
Suction irrigator	—
Advanced bipolar instrument	—
Monopolar laparoscopic shears	Power settings: 60 cut, 40 coagulation
Sutures	
0-Polyglactin 910 (Vicryl) on GU needle	Umbilical fascial closure
2–0 PDS on CT-1	Modified Richardson stitch on vaginal cuff pedicle
2–0 V-lock	Vaginal cuff running closure
Laparoscopic needle drivers	—
Tissue extraction bag	—

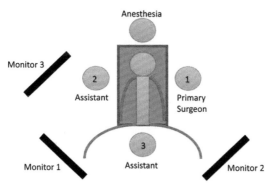

Fig. 1. Operating room setup.

decompression of gastric contents. The orogastric tube placement is pivotal if a left upper quadrant abdominal entry is anticipated.

Focus is next placed on positioning of the patients' lower extremities. The buttocks is brought down to the edge of the table to allow room for insertion and manipulation of the uterine manipulator. Patients are placed in the dorsal low lithotomy position, most commonly using Allen stirrups. Careful attention to pressure points must be prioritized to decrease occurrence of postoperative neuropathy. The two nerve bundles at highest risk of injury after laparoscopic hysterectomy include the common peroneal nerve and the femoral nerve. Nerve injuries are estimated to occur at a rate of 0.2% to 2.0% and are most commonly injured secondary to surgical positioning.[13]

The common peroneal nerve is at risk of compression during lower extremity positioning, specifically at the level of the fibular head.[13] This injury can occur if excessive pressure is placed between the lateral knee and the stirrup. The lower extremity should be positioned with the patients' ankle, knee, hip, and contralateral shoulder aligned. Symptoms of common peroneal neuropraxia include lateral foot paresthesia and foot drop. These symptoms commonly resolve on their own.

Femoral nerve injuries are also associated with incorrect lithotomy positioning. If the hip is placed in excessive flexion or the lower extremity is placed in excessive abduction and internal rotation, the femoral nerve can be compressed.[13] Femoral nerve injury may result in impaired hip flexion or knee extension. When positioning the stirrups it is imperative to limit hip flexion to less than 80° and monitor appropriate thigh abduction and rotation.

Bilateral tucking of the upper extremity is performed for all laparoscopic cases. It is important to maintain a neutral position when positioning the arms in attempt to optimize patient safety and decrease the risk of nerve injury. The brachial plexus and ulnar nerve are most at risk in gynecologic surgery; special attention should be placed on the shoulders, elbows, wrists, and hands.

Energy Sources

There are multiple energy sources available to assist in laparoscopic and vaginal dissection, including bipolar, monopolar, and harmonic energy. Many advanced instruments incorporate a combination of these energy options, in addition to cutting capabilities. The specific instruments used are often based on surgeon preference and institution availability.

The tissue effect of monopolar energy can be adjusted through the size of electrode, length of time energy is administered, timing of energy activation in relation to tissue contact, and cutting versus coagulation waveform. Various monopolar instruments include endoshears, a hook, or a spatula. Monopolar energy is particularly useful when creating the bladder flap as well as the colpotomy.

Advanced bipolar vessel sealing and cutting devices have become increasingly popular secondary to their enhanced sealing power and decreased thermal spread. Currently available models include the LigaSure (Medtronic, Minneapolis, MN), EnSeal (Ethicon, Somerville, NJ), Caiman (Aesculap Inc, Center Valley, PA), and PKS Cutting Forceps (Olympus, Center Valley, PA). Instruments that combine various energy modalities include the Thunderbeat from Olympus (Center Valley, PA), which includes both advanced bipolar and ultrasonic capabilities, as well as the LigaSure Advance (Medtronic, Minneapolis, MN), which includes both advanced bipolar and monopolar technologies. Regardless of the energy used, it is pivotal that the surgeon understands the fundamentals of electrosurgery to optimize the instrument's capabilities and minimize complications.

Approach

Technique/procedure (detailed steps)

Uterine manipulation Correct placement of a uterine manipulator and colpotomizer cup is essential in providing optimal uterine manipulation and identifying the correct colpotomy location. The uterine attachment of the uterosacral ligaments are often a reliable landmark in assessing cup location, as this junction is commonly the location of colpotomy for a total laparoscopic hysterectomy. The authors use the RUMI II uterine manipulator (Cooper Surgical, Trumbull, CT) as this provides various options for tip length and cervical cup size.

Laparoscopic entry Most laparoscopic complications occur with initial abdominal entry, which emphasizes the importance of obtaining a detailed surgical history and having a thorough knowledge of pelvic anatomy. Opinion continues to be divided as to the best and safest method of abdominal entry between the open and closed technique. A Cochrane review found that there was a reduction in the rate of failed entry with the use of an open technique; however, there was no difference between the open and closed techniques for vascular or visceral injuries. The choice of entry is commonly based on the surgeon's experience and comfort level with a specific method.

Initial entry is most commonly achieved at the umbilicus, as this is the thinnest portion of the anterior abdominal wall secondary to the fusion of the 3 fascial layers including the external oblique, internal oblique, and transversalis. Patients should be in the supine position during initial entry as Trendelenburg positioning can angle the great vessels anteriorly and increase the risk of vascular injury.

Multiple prior abdominal surgeries, umbilical mesh placement, or a large pelvic mass may warrant an alternate site for initial abdominal entry. In these clinical scenarios, the left upper quadrant at the Palmer point is often an excellent alternative. An orogastric tube should be inserted when the left upper quadrant is used to protect the stomach. Additional underlying structures that should be noted include the spleen, pancreas, and liver.

Once intraperitoneal access is confirmed, the pneumoperitoneum is increased to approximately 15 mm Hg. The area directly below entry should first be evaluated to ensure inadvertent injury of underlying bowel, bladder, or vasculature did not occur. Patients are then placed in Trendelenburg position, and accessory ports are placed under direct laparoscopic visualization. The course of the inferior epigastric vessels should be noted before placing lateral lower quadrant ports. If a suprapubic port is used, a Foley catheter should be placed before trocar insertion for adequate bladder decompression. If the upper margin of the bladder is difficult to identify, the bladder can be backfilled to assist with identifying the upper margin.

Round ligament transection The round ligament is first identified coursing toward the inguinal canal and is placed on upward traction. Using the uterine manipulator, the uterus is placed on traction toward the opposite sidewall and the avascular portion of the broad ligament is identified. The round ligament is transected lateral to the varicose vessels within the broad ligament to minimize bleeding (**Fig. 2**).

Bladder flap development Focus is next placed on development of the bladder flap. The uterus is kept in the midline to retroverted position with inward traction achieved with the assistance of the uterine manipulator. The assistant may also apply fundal pressure to assist with visualization of the anterior lower uterine segment. The colpotomy cup location is confirmed laparoscopically and serves as a guide for dissection. An atraumatic grasper is used to apply upward traction on the anterior leaf of the broad ligament, which allows carbon dioxide (CO_2) gas to assist in dissecting the vesicovaginal avascular plane. The peritoneum is then incised from the round ligament stump to the colpotomy cup and then curved upward toward the contralateral round ligament. The bladder is then mobilized off of the lower uterine segment. Using an atraumatic grasper, the bladder is held on upward tension toward the anterior abdominal wall and the vesicovaginal plane is identified (**Fig. 3**). Using both blunt and sharp dissection, the bladder is mobilized off of the colpotomizer cup. Dissection is focused midline on the cup, with lateral dissection completed with uterine artery skeletonization.

Ligating the cornual pedicles Regardless of ovarian retention or removal, a window is created in the avascular portion of the posterior leaf of the broad ligament whenever possible. This peritoneal window is developed superior to the ureter and extended bluntly parallel to the cervix (**Fig. 4**). This window assists in further skeletonizing the utero-ovarian ligament and infundibulopelvic (IP) ligament and ensures that the ureter is not included in this pedicle. When transecting the utero-ovarian ligament, the cornual region should be avoided to minimize uterine bleeding (**Fig. 5**). If an oophorectomy is being performed, the peritoneum parallel to the IP ligament is transected proximally to provide optimal skeletonization and visualization of the vessels in relation to the ureter. With the ureter in view, the IP ligament is then desiccated and transected. If the ovaries are to remain, a salpingectomy is typically performed at the conclusion of the case in attempt to optimize visualization during the hysterectomy.

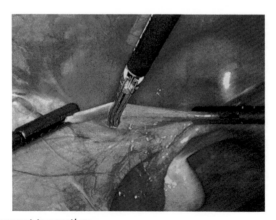

Fig. 2. Round ligament transection.

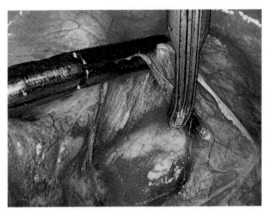

Fig. 3. Development of the bladder flap.

Uterine vessel skeletonization Before transecting the uterine vessels, adequate skeletonization is pivotal in providing optimal hemostasis and minimizing the risk of bladder, ureter, and bowel injury. Traction on the uterus should be maintained in a slightly anteverted orientation with inward pressure, which typically allows adequate visualization of the posterior cul-de-sac and uterosacral ligaments. The posterior leaf of the broad ligament is first dissected to the colpotomizer cup, which is often proximal to the uterosacral ligament uterine attachment (**Fig. 6**). This dissection assists in exposing the uterine vessels and further mobilizes the ureter laterally, away from the pedicle. The bladder is next examined anteriorly, and the lateral attachments are mobilized off of the lower uterine segment and uterine vessels. Finally, the areolar tissue that surrounds the uterine vessels should be divided and retracted caudally.

Securing the uterine artery Once the uterine vessels are adequately skeletonized, uterine artery desiccation and division can be safely executed. The uterus is kept on constant inward pressure, which assists in maximizing the distance between the uterine pedicle and ureter. A bipolar instrument or advanced vessel-sealing device is used to coagulate the uterine vessels at the level of the internal os (**Fig. 7**). The posterior peritoneum is not included in this pedicle to ensure that the ureter maintains a lateral position. The vessel-sealing instrument should bounce off the colpotomizer cup to ensure all vessels are being included, including the medial branches.

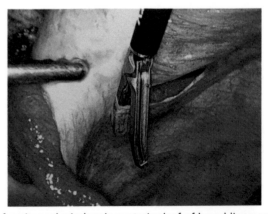

Fig. 4. Creation of peritoneal window in posterior leaf of broad ligament.

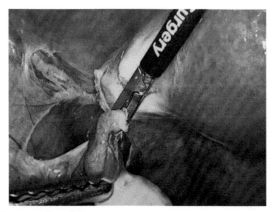

Fig. 5. Ligating the cornual pedicles.

Coagulation should be focused on tissue that is superior and medial to the colpotomy cup to minimize thermal injury to the ureter. Once transected, the pedicle should be mobilized inferior and lateral to the colpotomy cup to confirm the endopelvic fascia is absent of vessels.

Colpotomy The colpotomy can be created using a variety of techniques, including monopolar energy, bipolar energy, ultrasonic energy, or a cold knife. A correctly placed colpotomizer cup can assist in identifying the cervicovaginal junction and serve as a guide for circumferential transection. If a colpotomizer cup is unable to be inserted, alternate modalities can be used to delineate this margin, including Breisky-Navratil (Novosurgical, Oak Brooks, IL) vaginal retractors, a sponge stick, or infant suction bulb with the tip removed. The colpotomy can be started anteriorly or posteriorly and is carried around circumferentially with visualization optimized using strategic manipulation of the uterine manipulator (**Fig. 8**). Minimizing energy application during colpotomy enhances vascular blood flow to the vaginal cuff and promotes postoperative healing.

Once the cervix is adequately dissected from the vagina, the specimen is removed through the vagina or abdominally depending on the uterine size. For further discussion on uterine morcellation, please see Dr Barker MA: Current Issues with Hysterectomy, in this issue. The vagina is occluded with a glove containing a sponge to maintain pneumoperitoneum.

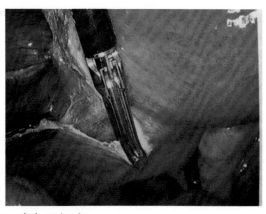

Fig. 6. Uterine artery skeletonization.

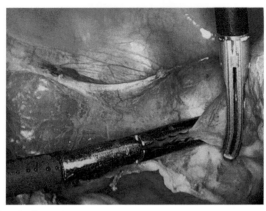

Fig. 7. Securing the uterine artery.

Vaginal cuff closure Meticulous surgical technique is necessary when closing the vaginal cuff laparoscopically to minimize postoperative complications, including hemorrhage and vaginal cuff dehiscence. Attention is first placed on the vaginal angles. A modified Richardson stitch is performed using a monofilament delayed absorbable suture, which incorporates the uterosacral ligament and compresses vessels medial to the uterine pedicle to further enhance hemostasis (**Fig. 9**). The angle stitches are tied with extracorporeal knots, which allows the elongated suture tails to be secured outside of the ipsilateral lower quadrant port. These stay sutures allow the cuff to be maintained on upward tension, which assists in delineating the anatomy and drops the bladder away from the vaginal cuff margin. The vaginal cuff is sutured in a transverse fashion, being certain to incorporate vaginal mucosa as well as pubocervical and rectovaginal fascia. Closure can be performed in a running fashion or with figure-of-8 or interrupted sutures, with approximately 1 cm between each stitch (**Figs. 10** and **11**).

VAGINAL ASSISTANCE TO LAPAROSCOPIC HYSTERECTOMY

The amount of vaginal surgery necessary depends on the indication for surgery and level of skill of the surgeon. The aforementioned steps in the laparoscopic section describe a hysterectomy top to bottom, whereas this section describes the steps

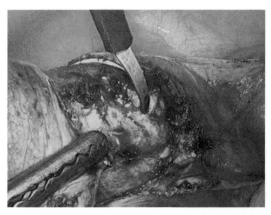

Fig. 8. Colpotomy

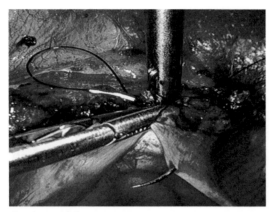

Fig. 9. Modified Richardson stitch.

bottom to top, concluding at the level of the utero-ovarian ligaments. The stirrups should be elevated to provide adequate visualization of the vagina.

Colpotomy

The cervix is grasped with a tenaculum at the 6- and 12-o'clock position. The authors prefer to inject a dilute vasopressin solution circumferentially around the cervix; however, this is left to surgeon preference. A scalpel is used to circumferentially incise the cervix down to the level of the pubocervical fascia. Electrocautery is used to maintain hemostasis. Scissors dissect the vesicouterine peritoneum and aid in entry into the anterior peritoneal cavity. Visual confirmation is obtained by either a rush of CO_2 gas from the laparoscopic portion of the procedure or by visualization of the bowel. A Deaver retractor is placed to elevate the bladder and ureters. The cervix is then elevated anteriorly, and the uterosacral ligaments are palpated and identified. Mayo scissors are used to sharply enter, and a retractor blade is placed in the posterior cul-de-sac.

Secure the Uterine Artery

Heaney clamps are used to secure the uterosacral ligaments bilaterally. They are cut and the suture is ligated with heavy absorbable suture (such as 0 polyglactin).

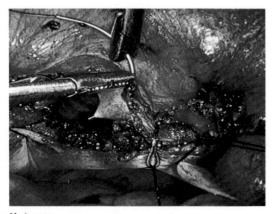

Fig. 10. Vaginal cuff closure.

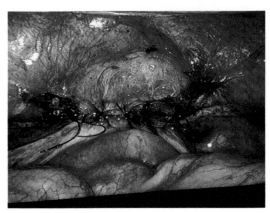

Fig. 11. Closed cuff.

Successive bites are taken to clamp, transect, and ligate the cardinal ligament complex up to and including the uterine vessels. Care is taken to avoid the ureters by upward traction on the Deaver retractor. Alternatively, instead of the traditional clamp, cut, and tie method, there are several handheld tissue-sealing devices that can be used in these steps. Assuming the utero-ovarian ligaments were managed laparoscopic, the uterus will be free from all connections and can be delivered through the vagina.

Vaginal Cuff Closure

If apical suspension sutures are indicated (prolapse), then placement of Mayo-McCall sutures are performed before cuff closure (See Occhino JA, Byrnes J: Hysterectomy for Benign Conditions of the Uterus: Total Vaginal Hysterectomy, in this issue). The cuff is closed horizontally using several interrupted sutures of heavy absorbable suture (such as 0 polyglactin) and usually requires 5 to 7 sutures. Angle sutures are placed first followed by interrupted suture to close the central aspect of the cuff. Cystourethroscopy is performed to ensure bilateral ureteral efflux. The addition of oral phenazopyridine hydrochloride (Pyridium) preoperatively aids in visualization.

COMPLICATIONS AND MANAGEMENT

Complications of hysterectomy vary based on route of hysterectomy, patient characteristics, surgeon experience, and operative technique. The most common complications after laparoscopic hysterectomy can be categorized as infectious, venous thromboembolic, hemorrhagic, nerve injury, genitourinary, gastrointestinal, and vaginal cuff dehiscence (**Table 4**).[13]

Bleeding

All patients should have a blood type and screen done before surgery. When bleeding is encountered, there are a variety of energy sources now available to assist in obtaining hemostasis. Before utilization of energy sources, adequate visualization of the bleeding source is key to prevent inadvertent damage to surrounding structures, such as the ureter and bowel. In addition, surgical clips are a resource.

Urinary Tract Injury

Genitourinary structures are damaged by sharp dissection, including transection as well as with energy (which can present as a delayed injury weeks after surgery) and

Table 4 Complications	
Complication	**Rate (%)**
Conversion to laparotomy	2.7–3.9
Infectious	9
Vaginal cuff cellulitis	
Infected hematoma	
Wound infection	
Urinary tract infection	
Respiratory infection	
Venous thromboembolic	1.0–2.9
Hemorrhagic	2.0–5.1
Nerve injury	0.2–2.0
Femoral	
Iliohypogastric and ilioinguinal	
Peroneal	
Genitourinary	1–2
Gastrointestinal	0.1–0.4
Vaginal cuff dehiscence	1–2

Data from Clarke-Pearson D, Geller E. Complications of hysterectomy. Obstet Gynecol 2013;121(3):654–73.

with suture placement. Tracing the course of the ureter in surgery is fundamental, but there are times when visualization is not optimal (eg, severe endometriosis or large fibroids). Although ureteral stent placement has not been shown to decrease the rate of injury, it may still be beneficial in some situations.[14] In addition, cystoscopy may be performed after hysterectomy to confirm patency of ureters at the time of surgery. This procedure will help identify ureteral transection and complete occlusion with suture placement but may not identify a partial transection or occlusion. Transections will require reapproximation or reimplantation and can be performed laparoscopically with the appropriately trained surgeon. Suture occlusions should be removed and the ureter stented for several weeks.

Bladder injuries will typically occur at the dome and can be repaired with a double-layered closure of absorbable sutures. Watertight integrity should be confirmed by backfilling the bladder and observing the repair via the laparoscope. If the injury is near the trigone, then ureteral stent placement is often performed before the closure of the injury. Cystoscopy should always be performed to ensure patency of the ureters. Postoperative catheter drainage is recommended, especially if damage occurred near the trigone or dependent portion of the bladder.

POSTOPERATIVE CARE

Standard care is performed in the immediate postoperative period. Patients are typically more mobile given the lack of a large abdominal incision; therefore, early ambulation is encouraged (**Table 5**). In select patients, same-day discharge is possible with appropriate preoperative counseling and hospital infrastructure. However, many patients will stay overnight (typically as a 23-hour observation). Once discharged, they are given the following instructions.

Table 5	
Postoperative care	
Ambulation	Remain mobile; limit time in bed to sleep only; no running or strenuous activities
Pain control	Ibuprofen and acetaminophen on a scheduled basis; addition of narcotic medication as needed
Diet	No restrictions
Pelvic rest	No lifting more than 10 lb for 6 wk; nothing in the vagina for at least 6 wk and postoperative pelvic examination
Skin care	Keep area clean and dry
Bowel regimen	Stool softeners while on narcotic medication

REPORTING, FOLLOW-UP, AND CLINICAL IMPLICATIONS

Patients are seen at the 4- to 6-week postoperative visit for evaluation; but no long-term follow-up is typically indicated, and patients will return only as needed. They should undergo routine pelvic examinations by their provider, and Papanicolaou test guidelines should be followed as indicated. Vaginal cuff dehiscence has been reported in laparoscopic hysterectomies.[15] Thorough examination of the vaginal cuff should be performed before patients can resume intercourse. Cases have been reported greater than 12 months after hysterectomy; therefore, any patient complaint that may suggest disruption of the cuff should be evaluated.[13]

OUTCOMES

Laparoscopic hysterectomy has historically been associated with an increased risk of urinary tract injury; however, a recent systematic review estimated the frequency at 0.73%, which is comparable with abdominal hysterectomy.[16] Vaginal cuff dehiscence can occur (1.35%) in total laparoscopic hysterectomy and (0.28%) in laparoscopic-assisted vaginal hysterectomy compared with 0.15% in abdominal and 0.08% in vaginal.[17] A Cochrane review showed no difference by laparoscopic hysterectomy and abdominal hysterectomy in terms of primary outcomes (satisfaction, quality of life, intraoperative visceral injury, and major long-term complications) but did show a quicker return to normal activity and an increased risk of urinary tract injury with laparoscopic hysterectomy.[18]

CURRENT CONTROVERSIES/FUTURE CONSIDERATIONS

The main controversy with total laparoscopic hysterectomy/laparoscopic-assisted vaginal hysterectomy is adequate training. A recent Canadian study of graduating residents showed that only 26% felt comfortable performing a total laparoscopic hysterectomy and 63.4% with a laparoscopic-assisted vaginal hysterectomy.[19] This finding compares with a recent study revealing 22% of US residents feeling completely prepared to perform a laparoscopic hysterectomy and 28% for a vaginal hysterectomy.[20] Advanced training in one of the several gynecology fellowships is an option for increased training.

SUMMARY

1. When vaginal hysterectomy is not possible, laparoscopic hysterectomy and laparoscopic-assisted vaginal hysterectomy are excellent methods for removal of the uterus.

2. Poor uterine descent and need to evaluate the pelvis are examples of indications for use of laparoscopy with performance of hysterectomy.
3. Advanced laparoscopic skills are often required to complete a total laparoscopic hysterectomy. Completion of the hysterectomy vaginally is an option, with the amount of vaginal dissection required dependent on the laparoscopic portion.
4. Cystoscopy is recommended after all hysterectomies.
5. Patients will return to work sooner with decreased pain and a shorter hospital stay when compared with those who undergo abdominal hysterectomy.

REFERENCES

1. Sutton C. Hysterectomy: a historical perspective. Baillieres Clin Obstet Gynaecol 1997;11(1):1–22.
2. Moen MD, Richter HE. Vaginal hysterectomy: past, present, and future. Int Urogynecol J 2014;25:1161–5.
3. Reich H, DeCaprio J, McGlynn F. Laparoscopy hysterectomy. J Gynecol Surg 1989;5:13–215.
4. Kovac SR, Cruikshank SH, Retto H. Laparoscopy-assisted vaginal hysterectomy. J Gynecol Surg 1990;6:185–93.
5. Munro MG, Parker WH. A classification system for laparoscopic hysterectomy. Obstet Gynecol 1993;82(4 Pt 1):624–9.
6. Wright JD, Herzog TJ, Tsui J, et al. Nationwide trends in the performance of inpatient hysterectomy in the United States. Obstet Gynecol 2013;122:233–41.
7. Reich H. Total laparoscopic hysterectomy: indications, techniques and outcomes. Curr Opin Obstet Gynecol 2007;19:337–44.
8. AAGL Advancing Minimally Invasive Gynecology Worldwide. AAGL position statement: route of hysterectomy to treat benign uterine disease. J Minim Invasive Gynecol 2011;18(1):1–3.
9. Muzii L, Angioli R, Zullo MA, et al. Bowel preparation for gynecological surgery. Crit Rev Oncol Hematol 2003;48:311–5.
10. Fanning J, Valea F. Perioperative bowel management for gynecologic surgery. Am J Obstet Gynecol 2011;205(4):309–14.
11. Guenaga KK, Matos D, Castro AA, et al. Mechanical bowel preparation for elective colorectal surgery. Cochrane Database Syst Rev 2005;(1):CD001544.
12. Yang L, Arden D, Lee T, et al. Mechanical bowel preparation for gynecologic laparoscopy: a prospective randomized trial of oral sodium phosphate solution vs single sodium phosphate enema. J Minim Invasive Gynecol 2011; 18:149–56.
13. Clarke-Pearson D, Geller E. Complications of hysterectomy. Obstet Gynecol 2013;121(3):654–73.
14. Chou MT, Wang CJ, Lien RC. Prophylactic ureteral catheterization in gynecologic surgery: a 12-year randomized trial in a community hospital. Int Urogynecol J 2009;20:689–93.
15. Hur HC, Donnellan N, Mansuria S, et al. Vaginal cuff dehiscence after different modes of hysterectomy. Obstet Gynecol 2011;118(4):794–801.
16. Adelman MR, Bardsley TR, Sharp HT. Urinary tract injuries in laparoscopic hysterectomy: a systematic review. J Minim Invasive Gynecol 2014;21(4):558–66.
17. Uccella S, Ghezzi F, Mariani A, et al. Vaginal cuff closure after minimally invasive hysterectomy: our experience and systematic review of the literature. Am J Obstet Gynecol 2011;205:119.e1-12.

18. Aarts JW, Nieboer TE, Johnson N, et al. Surgical approach to hysterectomy for benign gynaecological disease. Cochrane Database Syst Rev 2015;(8):CD003677.
19. Kroft J, Moody JRK, Lee P. Canadian hysterectomy educational experience: survey of recent graduates in obstetrics and gynecology. J Minim Invasive Gynecol 2011;18:438–44.
20. Burkett D, Horwitz J, Kennedy V, et al. Assessing current trends in resident hysterectomy training. Female Pelvic Med Reconstr Surg 2011;17:210–4.

The Essential Elements of a Robotic-Assisted Laparoscopic Hysterectomy

Khara M. Simpson, MD[a], Arnold P. Advincula, MD[b],*

KEYWORDS

- Robotics • Laparoscopy • Hysterectomy • Minimally invasive surgery

KEY POINTS

- A successful robotic-assisted laparoscopic hysterectomy starts with choosing the right patient and having the appropriate operating room set up with special attention paid to proper patient positioning.
- Identification and isolation of relevant anatomy, appropriate placement of the Koh colpotomy cup, and cephalad traction of the uterus are paramount in preventing organ injury.
- Maintaining meticulous hemostasis throughout the procedure with the judicious use of energy and proper pedicle formation is essential to reducing blood loss.
- Same-day discharge is safe and cost-effective following uncomplicated procedures.
- Perioperative outcomes are similar to laparoscopic hysterectomy with the exclusion of operative time, which may lead to increased costs.

 Video content accompanies this article at http://www.obgyn.theclinics.com.

INTRODUCTION

Robotics entered the surgical arena in a formal way in the mid-1980s with a primary goal of improving surgeon precision and accuracy. This goal led to the development of a device to assist neurosurgeons with stereotactic biopsies.[1–3] From there, several different models were created for specialty-specific procedures with the greatest penetration in orthopedics. It was the merging of robotics and virtual reality, however,

Financial Disclosures: Nothing to disclose (K.M. Simpson); Blue Endo, Cooper Surgical, Intuitive Surgical, Titan Medical (A.P. Advincula).
[a] Gynecologic Specialty Surgery, Department of Obstetrics and Gynecology, Columbia University Medical Center, 622 West 168th Street, PH 16, Room 127, New York, NY 10032, USA;
[b] Department of Obstetrics and Gynecology, Sloane Hospital for Women, Simulation Center, Columbia University Medical Center, New York-Presbyterian Hospital, 622 West 168th Street, PH 16, Room 127, New York, NY 10032, USA
* Corresponding author.
E-mail address: aa3530@cumc.columbia.edu

Obstet Gynecol Clin N Am 43 (2016) 479–493
http://dx.doi.org/10.1016/j.ogc.2016.04.008
0889-8545/16/$ – see front matter © 2016 Elsevier Inc. All rights reserved.

obgyn.theclinics.com

that led to the precursors of modern-day systems. The National Aeronautics and Space Administration and the Stanford Research Institute were key contributors in the creation of virtual reality environments and the concept of telepresence. These concepts were rapidly extrapolated to other industries, such as medicine, with significant potential seen in the expansion of surgeon skill set. The US Department of Defense took a keen interest in this dual technology and the possibility of telesurgery or remotely performed surgery during warfare. At their charge, continued technological advancements led to the introduction of the da Vinci Surgical System (Intuitive Surgical, Inc, Sunnyvale, CA, USA) in 1997 with the performance of the first robot-assisted laparoscopic cholecystectomy. Despite earlier plans for military applications, the device became integrated into routine clinical care for cardiac and urologic surgery.

Currently, the da Vinci Surgical System is the only robotic system that is approved by the US Food and Drug Administration (FDA) for laparoscopic procedures in general surgery, cardiac, colorectal, head and neck, thoracic, urologic, and gynecologic procedures. It was initially approved in 2000 for general laparoscopic use, and as of April 2005, was given FDA clearance for use in gynecologic procedures. The system consists of a surgeon's console, a mobile patient side cart with 3 or 4 robotic arms, and a video tower. A variety of multiuse Endowrist instruments are available, including needle drivers, graspers, energized instruments, and staplers. Three models currently exist, the Si–e (2 arms), the Si, and the newest version, the Xi System, which was released in 2015. The Xi system affords the opportunity for multiquadrant surgery via a new patient–side cart orientation, a computerized docking assistant, and the ability to use the camera from all ports. Surgeon training tools have been incorporated directly into the device. Intuitive Surgical reports there are approximately 2400 units in the United States and that gynecology is the leading specialty user of the device with 263,000 hysterectomies being performed robotically in the United States in 2015.[4]

Hysterectomy continues to be the most common major surgical procedure performed by gynecologists in the United States. Data from 2000 to 2004 suggest that greater than 600,000 procedures were performed every year with approximately two-thirds being performed abdominally for benign indications.[5] Despite the introduction of laparoscopy in the late 1990s, the vast majority of hysterectomies in 2009 for benign indications were still performed via the abdominal approach (56%) as compared with minimally invasive techniques such as conventional laparoscopy (20%).[6] One proposed obstacle to the more widespread acceptance and application of minimally invasive surgical techniques in gynecologic surgery has been the steep learning curve for surgeons. Other obstacles are the potential technical limitations of conventional laparoscopic instruments that include counterintuitive hand movements (fulcrum effect), an unsteady 2-dimensional visual field, and limited degrees of instrument motion within the body as well as ergonomic difficulty and tremor amplification.[3] Robotics may offer a solution with 3-dimensional vision, wristed instrumentation mirroring open surgical technique, and tremor dampening, leading to a quicker uptake of the technology. Wright and colleagues[7] noted this trend toward robotics with the analysis of inpatient rates of hysterectomy between 1998 and 2010, as shown in **Fig. 1**. Between 2002 and 2010, there was a 36.4% decrease in the overall rate of hysterectomy, which translated to decreases in abdominal and vaginal hysterectomies, a relatively stable number of laparoscopic hysterectomies, and an increase in robotic procedures.

Despite its documented advantages, robotics requires alternative laparoscopic port placement, lacks tactile feedback (haptics), and is reliant on a bedside assistant because the primary surgeon is positioned remote from the patient, necessitating

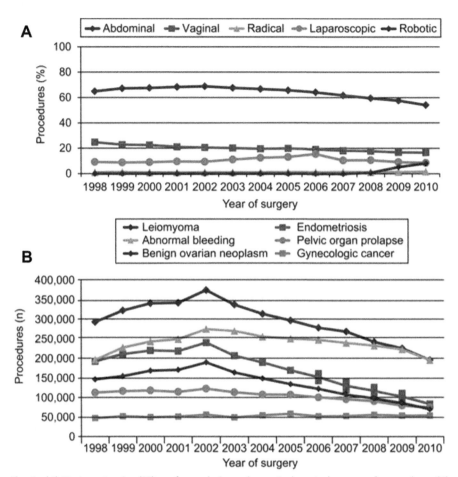

Fig. 1. (A) Hysterectomies (%) performed via each surgical route by year of procedure. (B) Procedures (n) performed each year stratified by indication for surgery. (From Wright J, Herzog T, Tsui J, et al. Nationwide trends in the performance of inpatient hysterectomy in the United States. Obstet Gynecol 2013;122(2 Pt 1):237; with permission.)

device-specific training to allow for successful application of this surgical tool and to prevent complications. The purpose of this article is to share key considerations for optimizing a robotic-assisted laparoscopic hysterectomy as well as a step-by-step technique (Video 1). A brief review of perioperative outcomes is also undertaken.

PREOPERATIVE EVALUATION

Hysterectomy represents definitive surgical management for a variety of benign and malignant indications, including symptomatic uterine fibroids and abnormal uterine bleeding. It also serves a role in the reduction of pelvic pain and symptoms related to endometriosis. It is commonly reserved for patients who have completed child-bearing or who have failed medical management or other conservative measures. The American Congress of Obstetricians and Gynecologists (ACOG) and the Society of Gynecologic Surgery Committee Opinion on robotic surgery in gynecology states that robot-assisted cases should be appropriately selected based on available data and expert opinion and that vaginal hysterectomy should be performed when feasible.[8] American Association of Gynecologic Laparoscopists supports a similar practice and emphasizes that robotics should not replace vaginal or laparoscopic hysterectomy when possible.[9] It is the authors' practice to approach smaller uteri without significant adhesive disease by a vaginal or conventional laparoscopic technique. A robotic-assisted laparoscopic approach is typically used with larger and/or distorted abnormalities or in anticipation of significant pelvic adhesive disease (ie, advanced endometriosis, patient history of uterine artery embolization, prior myomectomies or pelvic infections/abscesses) where finer dissection is required. The authors do not support a hard cutoff for uterine size above which a robotic approach should not be used. Specimens that preclude the performance of a robotic procedure include abnormality that approaches the costal margins preventing safe port placement, a broad lower uterine segment that compresses the pelvic sidewalls or obscures critical landmarks, and any significant concern for malignancy. The physical examination is critical in anticipating intra-abdominal abnormalities. Key components include identifying the upper extent of the uterus, the width of the uterus as defined as the proximity to the pelvic sidewalls, and assessment of mobility as a proxy for pelvic adhesive disease.

All patients receive endometrial sampling before hysterectomy either via endometrial biopsy performed in the office, or for some low-risk patients, a dilation and curettage with frozen section at the beginning of the operative case. Patients with a significant fibroid burden and age greater than 50 may have total lactate dehydrogenase and isoenzymes drawn as well as an MRI for sarcoma evaluation similar to that reported by Goto and colleagues.[10] Preoperative laboratory tests are drawn in accordance with hospital policy based on a detailed patient questionnaire.

INTRAOPERATIVE SETUP

The first key component of surgery is appropriate operating room setup. This setup includes ensuring the desired equipment has been secured and is functional. This setup along with patient positioning, appropriate port placement (to avoid arm collisions), and robotic docking (to allow for pelvic access) can significantly impact the surgeon before starting the intra-abdominal portion of the case. The authors administer antibiotics according to ACOG guidelines[11] and venous thromboembolism prophylaxis according to hospital policy that recommends chemoprophylaxis more broadly than the ACOG guidelines.

Patient Positioning

Antiskid measures should be incorporated at the time of patient positioning, with a foam egg crate mattress pad directly behind the patient's upper back in order to avoid patient slippage during the use of Trendelenburg.[12,13] The authors use the Pink Pad (Xodus Medical, New Kensington, PA, USA), which is a multiunit system with memory foam padding along the back and arms as well as a padded chest strap.[14] All patients are placed in low dorsal lithotomy position with arms padded and tucked at their sides after general endotracheal anesthesia has been administered (**Fig. 2**). To avoid neuropathies, hip flexion should limited to a maximum of 170°; thigh abduction should be less than or equal to 90° with minimal external rotation. An examination under anesthesia is then performed with special attention paid to the shape and mobility of the uterus. This examination also allows for the planning of safe and functional port placement. The patient is then prepared and draped in the usual sterile fashion.

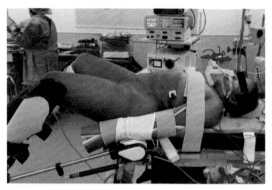

Fig. 2. Low-lithotomy patient positioning.

The bladder is drained with a Foley catheter, and the stomach is evacuated with an orogastric tube. Based on surgeon preference, a variety of uterine manipulators can then be placed in order to facilitate the robot-assisted hysterectomy. The authors use the reusable Advincula Arch in conjunction with an RUMI tip, Koh colpotomy cup, and vaginal pneumo-occluder balloon, or the disposable Advincula delineator (**Fig. 3**) that incorporates all pieces into one device (Cooper Surgical, Trumbull, CT, USA). Care should be taken to choose the right size cup for the specimen. Poorly placed or inappropriately sized colpotomy cups can make delineation of the cervico-vaginal junction difficult, causing excessive resection of the vagina or potential injury to the adjacent ureters or bladder.

Port Placement

Pneumoperitoneum is typically obtained with a Veress needle technique at the umbilicus, followed by placement of either 4 or 5 trocars, depending on the complexity of the case and a need for the fourth robotic arm. Intra-abdominal pressure is maintained at 20 mm Hg during port placement and then lowered to 15 mm Hg. The authors use a 3-armed patient side cart with the accessory port placed on the patient's right side (**Fig. 4**). **Fig. 5** illustrates the use of a 4-armed patient side cart setup. Depending on where the fourth arm is placed, the accessory port and bedside assistant are placed on the opposite side.

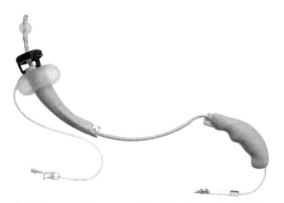

Fig. 3. The Advincula Delineator. (Image provided by CooperSurgical Inc., Trumbull, CT.)

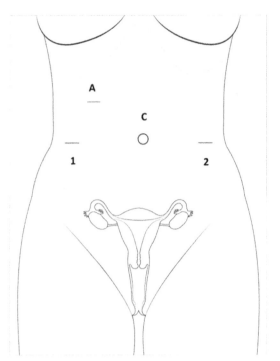

Fig. 4. Three-arm robotic setup: (A) 5-mm accessory port. (C) 12-mm camera port. (1) 8-mm robotic port, monopolar shears. (2) 8-mm robotic port, PK Dissector. (*Courtesy of* Columbia University, New York, NY; with permission.)

Immediately following insufflation, a 5-mm AirSeal (SurgiQuest, Milford, CT, USA) accessory port is optically placed, in the right upper quadrant in the midclavicular line, 2 to 3 fingerbreadths below the costal margin. AirSeal technology ensures a stable pneumoperitoneum and constant smoke evacuation. The abdominal cavity is surveyed to confirm case feasibility and to rule out any potential injuries during peritoneal access. A long, 12-mm nonrobotic port is then placed at the umbilicus. This port accommodates the dual optical endoscope. Camera placement at the umbilicus is useful for most uteri regardless of size because the focal point is the lower uterine segment and cervix. As a general rule, a handbreadth or approximately 8 to 10 cm between the endoscope and the focal point during uterine manipulation is necessary in order to allow for an adequate working distance. Two 8-mm robotic ports are placed in the left and right lower quadrants, respectively. These ports are located 2 fingerbreadths medial to the anterior-superior iliac spines at the lower level of the umbilicus, as seen in **Fig. 5**. For smaller uteri, these landmarks can be moved caudad. If the fourth robotic arm is used, the port will mirror the assistant port on the patient's left side. Once all desired ports are in place, the patient is placed in the Trendelenburg position. The goals of Trendelenburg are to fully visualize the Koh cup and for cephalad retraction of the large bowel. Small bowel may be placed in the right upper quadrant laparoscopically before docking. Routine "steep" Trendelenburg is avoided because lower angles have been shown to be effective for the performance of gynecologic robotic procedures.[15]

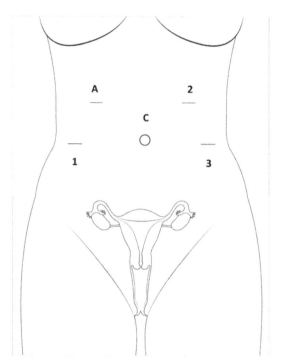

Fig. 5. Four-arm robotic setup. (A) 5-mm accessory port. (C) 12-mm camera port. (1) 8-mm robotic port, monopolar shears. (2) 8-mm robotic port, PK Dissector. (3) 8-mm robotic port, third arm, ProGrasp or Tenaculum. Note the difference in location of the 2 and 3 arms compared with the 3-arm setup. (*Courtesy of* Columbia University, New York, NY; with permission.)

Robotic Docking/Instrumentation

The robotic system can be either center or side docked. The authors prefer side docking to allow pelvic access for uterine manipulation and tissue extraction. The patient side cart is typically patient left-side docked. The left leg of the patient side cart should be oriented at a 45° angle with the left corner of the bed directed toward the patient's right shoulder. Each port is attached to the assigned robotic arm, with the exception of the accessory port, as shown in **Figs. 4** and **5**.

Each case begins with bipolar PK dissecting forceps on the surgeon's left (arm 2) and monopolar Hot Shears on the surgeon's right (arm 3). The monopolar current provided to the Hot Shears is kept to a minimum at 35 for both coagulation and cut functions. Factory default settings on the Gyrus ACMI generator are used for the bipolar PK dissecting forceps.

STEPS OF THE PROCEDURE

Key points

- A tension-free technique should be used with transection of vascular pedicles.
- Sealing vascular pedicles proximal to the uterus prevents back bleeding from ascending branches of the uterine vessels. Ensuring adequate pedicles on both the patient and the specimen side will further reduce bleeding.
- Tissue should not be transected beyond the area of dissection to prevent injury.

- Any form of energy should be applied judiciously.
- Upward tension on the uterine manipulator and Koh colpotomy cup from below are essential to defining anatomic landmarks and lateralizing the ureters.

Anatomic Survey

Careful attention must be paid to ensure that the ureters are identified bilaterally, and their relationship to the uterine vessels is noted. It is also desirable to visualize the Koh colpotomy cup anteriorly and posteriorly.

Ovarian Conservation

Regardless of whether the adnexa are going to be removed in conjunction with the hysterectomy, the adnexa are initially detached from the uterus in order to avoid both an obstructed view of the broad ligament and unnecessary retraction by the bedside assistant. With adnexal conservation, the utero-ovarian ligament and tube are sealed and transected proximally. The remainder of the salpingectomy is performed with transection of the mesosalpinx to the distal end of the tube. The fallopian tubes may also be removed following completion of the hysterectomy.

Risk-reducing salpingectomies are performed in accordance with the Society of Gynecologic Oncology clinical practice statement to consider salpingectomy at the time of pelvic surgery to reduce the risk of ovarian cancer.[16] Care must be taken however to avoid disruption of the infundibulopelvic ligament. Hysterectomy alone with complete adnexal conservation reduces the interval to menopause by up to 4 years, and added salpingectomy may reduce that interval further.[17]

If adnexa are to be removed as part of the hysterectomy, this can be accomplished before colpotomy, with specimens placed in the posterior cul-de-sac for retrieval after delivery of the uterus into the vagina. After proper skeletonization of the infundibulo-pelvic ligaments and identification of the ureters in the retroperitoneum bilaterally, the bipolar PK dissecting forceps are used to coagulate and seal these vascular pedicles, followed by transection with the monopolar Hot Shears. A tension-free technique is critical to successful ligation of the pedicle.

Transection of the Round Ligament

From the area of transection of the utero-ovarian ligament and the fallopian tube, the round ligaments are identified, coagulated, and transected laterally, approximately one-third away from the uterine body to avoid bleeding from the ascending branches of the uterine vessels. This provides access to the broad ligament for further dissection of the anterior and posterior leaves.

Broad Ligament Dissection

The anterior and posterior leaves are separated with blunt dissection. The Koh colpotomy cup should be identified, and dissection of the broad ligament should occur in the direction of the beveled edge of the cup. The surgical assistant should be applying upward pressure on the uterus to distance the uterine corpus and the surrounding broad ligament away from the bladder. One must be mindful of the location of the bladder and the uterine vessels during dissection. This portion of the procedure may be performed with hot or cold scissors. Anteriorly, the tissue is elevated with the PK Dissector, and if clear, transected with the monopolar Hot Shears. If fat is encountered during dissection, the bladder may be near, and a more cephalad transection of the broad ligament should be performed. The uterus is then anteverted to perform the posterior dissection. In a similar fashion, the broad ligament is deflected downward, away from the uterus and transected once deemed clear. Again, dissection is in the direction of the Koh colpotomy cup. This part of the dissection is essential in lateralizing the ureter away from the uterine vessels at the point where dessication and transection will occur.

Bladder Flap Development

The broad ligament dissection is then continued in the midline along the vesicouterine reflection to create the bladder flap. The dissection is facilitated by cephalad uterine movement that is provided by the bedside assistant on the uterine manipulator. Alternatively, a fourth arm configuration allows the introduction of either a Tenaculum forceps or ProGrasp forceps for upward uterine traction. These steps allow the Koh colpotomy ring to become clearly delineated as a dissection landmark and for the ureters to be identified and fall laterally well out of harm's way. Creation of the vesicouterine reflection should reveal the shiny and white tissue of the pubocervical fascia while simultaneously better defining the appearance of the colpotomy ring.

Skeletonization and Transection of Uterine Vessels

Proper bilateral skeletonization of the uterine vascular pedicle will allow for a much better tissue effect from the radiofrequency current applied through the bipolar PK dissecting forceps and minimize any risk of lateral thermal spread to adjacent structures, such as the ureter and bladder. This technique of vascular pedicle skeletonization before ligation is consistent with that seen in an open hysterectomy. Areolar tissue surrounding the uterine vessels is elevated and transected. A tension-free application of the bipolar PK dissecting forceps is used during coagulation and dessication of the uterine vasculature at the level of the internal cervical os. Should the surgeon find it necessary to perform multiple applications, this must be balanced with the risk of excessive instrument and tissue heating, with possible lateral thermal spread to critical adjacent structures. Once the uterine vasculature is coagulated bilaterally, the uterus should become ischemic in appearance. When both sides of the hysterectomy have been performed and the bladder is sufficiently dissected away from the Koh colpotomy cup, the vessels are transected at a right angle to prevent shearing of the vessel. The vessel is then lateralized below the level of the cup to allow for the colpotomy. Care must be taken not to lateralize the uterine vessels too much because the ureters often run within 1.5 to 2 cm of the internal cervical os.[18]

Colpotomy/Specimen Removal/Vaginal Cuff Closure

In cases where a total laparoscopic hysterectomy is intended, the monopolar Hot Shears are used to divide the cardinal and uterosacral ligament complexes bilaterally in a manner consistent with an intrafascial hysterectomy. Pneumoperitoneum is maintained by inflation of the vaginal pneumo-occluder balloon placed at the onset of the case. Completion of both the anterior and the posterior colpotomy is facilitated by the Koh colpotomy ring, while upward uterine traction is provided by the bedside assistant. Cut or coagulation functions are acceptable for this portion of the procedure, and most importantly, dwell time should be minimized. Care should be taken not to devascularize the cuff to prevent the risk of vaginal cuff dehiscence.

Once the uterus and cervix are completely detached, the specimen, with or without adnexa, is delivered into the vagina. In cases where the uterus is too large to pass through the colpotomy incision, a manual cold knife tissue extraction technique can be used to debulk the specimen after containment and can be performed vaginally or abdominally. Abdominally, this technique is performed through a 3-cm extended umbilical incision. The authors use the ExCITE technique using concentric "c" incisions with a scalpel to divide the tissue in a fashion similar to the power morcellator.

The pneumo-occluder balloon can be replaced to maintain pneumoperitoneum during the closure of the vaginal cuff. A sterile glove stuffed with Ray-Tecs may also be used. A 12-inch 2-0 V-Loc-180 barbed suture (Medtronic, Minneapolis, MN, USA) on a GS21 needle is used to reapproximate the vaginal cuff. Care must be taken to ensure that adequate bites are taken far enough back from the cut edge of the vaginal cuff, where radiofrequency current was applied, in order to avoid a pull-through of suture and potentially a vaginal cuff dehiscence. Bites at the angles should incorporate the uterosacral ligament. At the conclusion of the vaginal cuff closure, the barbed suture should be cut flush with the tissue to avoid potential injury from adherence of the bowel, omentum, or bladder to a long suture tail following abdominal desufflation. During vaginal cuff closure, the Cobra grasper and the Mega Needle Driver are used. These 2 Endowrist instruments are placed in the left (arm 2) and right (arm 1) robotic arms, respectively. Alternatively, based on surgeon preference, the PK dissecting forceps can remain in place to help facilitate vaginal cuff closure. Once the vaginal cuff is closed, the pneumo-occlusive device is removed and the vaginal vault is inspected.

In cases where a laparoscopic subtotal hysterectomy is intended, the monopolar Hot Shears are used to amputate the uterine corpus below the internal os, followed by extraction of the specimen through an extended umbilical incision as mentioned earlier. The cervical stump can either be left open if hemostatic or closed with interrupted sutures of 0-Vicryl on CT-2 needles cut to 6 inches. The endocervical canal should be fulgurated to reduce the risk of cervical stump bleeding. The extent of the surgical dissection for supracervical hysterectomies is unchanged from a total hysterectomy. The only difference is the site of specimen transection. An adequate bladder flap as well as development of the broad ligament is critical to prevent injury to the bladder and ureters.

Before the conclusion of the procedure, all operative sites are irrigated, and a low insufflation pressure check (8 mm Hg) is performed to ensure hemostasis. All instruments are then removed; the robot is undocked, and pneumoperitoneum is released. Universal cystoscopy with mannitol is routinely performed. Port sites are closed accordingly.

POSTOPERATIVE CARE

Same day discharge, defined as observation less than 24 hours, has been reported in the literature for laparoscopic hysterectomy, as a safe and cost-effective method of discharge planning. Schiavone and colleagues[19] in 2012 noted 46% of laparoscopic hysterectomy patients underwent same day discharges in 2010 as compared with 11% in 2000. Re-evaluation and readmission rates were low, ranging from 3% to 4% but were slightly higher when compared with patients admitted for greater than 24 hours. Findings have been similar following robotic hysterectomy for both benign and malignant indications. Lee and colleagues[20] were able to achieve a 78% same-day discharge rate (defined as discharge directly from the postanesthesia care unit [PACU]) with 30-day readmission rates of 2.5%. Longer operative times, higher estimated blood loss (EBL), and cases concluding after 6 PM were risk factors for admission.

For these reasons, the authors' patients are offered same-day discharge barring no significant complications. A select portion also undergoes outpatient hysterectomy with discharge 4 to 6 hours after surgery. This discharge represents a collaborative effort between the surgeons, anesthesiologists, and PACU staff. Patients receive short-acting opiates, ketorolac, and antiemetics intraoperatively. Transverse abdominis plane blocks are intermittently used as well before the start of the operation. Following surgery, patients are advanced to regular diet and receive oral pain medications. Chemical or mechanical deep vein thrombosis prophylaxis is administered according to hospital policy if admitted. Patient-controlled analgesia is rare.

OUTCOMES

Outcomes of robotic surgery when compared with conventional laparoscopy have been varied. Most of the literature published is retrospective in nature and represents surgeons' early experiences with the device. The overwhelming amount of evidence however supports similar outcomes between the 2 modalities with the exclusion of operative time. Operative times were increased by 25 to 80 minutes depending on the cited source.[21–26] Perioperative complications, EBL, length of stay (LOS), and conversion rates tended to be similar to laparoscopic hysterectomy with a slight trend toward lower EBL and shorter LOS in the robotic cohorts.[22–26] In the most recent *Cochrane Review* by Liu and colleagues,[27] these findings remained true with robotic cases being approximately 42 minutes longer but with a shorter LOS of approximately 7 hours. The review included 4 randomized controlled trials (Green 2013; Lonnerfors 2014; Paraiso 2013; Sarlos 2010) with 371 women comparing robotic-assisted hysterectomy to laparoscopic hysterectomy or vaginal hysterectomy. Pooled data revealed no significant differences in intraoperative injury, bleeding, infection, conversion rates, quality of life, pain, reintervention, or readmission. The data however were of low- to moderate-quality evidence due to inconsistencies across the studies so no definitive conclusions regarding superiority could be established. Similar findings were noted in a recent meta-analysis by Albright and colleagues.[28] When robotic surgical experience was documented, the completed case totals before the start of the trials were 20, 30, and 49 cases. Interestingly, the literature regarding robotic learning curves reports a range from 20 to 90 cases.[29–31]

COMPLICATIONS

As noted earlier, several studies have compared the outcomes of robotic hysterectomy with laparoscopic hysterectomy with notably similar outcomes with organ injury, infection, and vaginal cuff dehiscence.[22–26] There is some suggestion that robotic hysterectomy is associated with a slightly higher rate of urinary tract infection and urinary retention,[22,32] but this has been inconsistent. Vaginal cuff dehiscence rates have ranged from less than 1% to 4% and are on par with conventional laparoscopic hysterectomy rates.[33–35]

FUTURE CONSIDERATIONS/CONTROVERSY

Central to all discussions regarding the integration of robotics into routine care is cost. Units range in price from $1.6 to $2 million and require an annual maintenance contract. Instruments are multiuse and cost between $500 and $600 per use. To amortize the robot over 7 years, approximately $200,000 per year per robot must be included in the cost of the surgical department with an additional $500 to $1000 per case to cover annual maintenance costs.[36]

Excluding the initial capital investment, increases in cost with robotic surgery are commonly associated with significant differences in operating room time and/or surgical supply costs.[36–40] Increases in the cost of robotic hysterectomy as compared with laparoscopic approaches range from $1700 to $2600 with maintenance fees included.[37,41,42] The extent to which costs are elevated however is variable because they can decrease with increasing hospital and surgeon volume. Wright and colleagues[41] report an increase in cost of $1700 over conventional laparoscopic hysterectomy that decreased to $700 when surgeon case numbers exceeded 50. This amount reflects current knowledge of learning curves with robotic hysterectomy and decreasing operative times with increased surgical experience.

SUMMARY

Robotics has been integrated into gynecology resources because it confers certain advantages over laparoscopy with improved surgeon ergonomics and wristed instrumentation and similar perioperative outcomes. For these reasons, robotics has been postulated to allow more complex cases to be performed minimally invasively, thereby decreasing the rate of abdominal surgery and associated complications.[22,25,43,44] Although reports are varied, it appears in high-volume centers that the robotic approach is comparable in cost to abdominal hysterectomy and still provides the benefits of reduced EBL, LOS, and improved quality of life.[45] The robotics learning curve may also be less than that of laparoscopy leading to a greater uptake. These benefits are supported in the literature because inpatient robotic and laparoscopic hysterectomy numbers are similar despite an almost 20-year difference in introduction.[7]

Despite its many advantages, robotic hysterectomy is often associated with longer operative times and resultant increased costs; this has served as a barrier to full adoption of the technology. In an era of value-based care, cost containment with optimal patient outcomes is critical. Technology that offers a potential reduction in the rate of open surgery and related complications warrants further investigation outside of cost analysis so as to not prematurely prevent a promising technology from being used. There is a strong need for prospective collection of data from expert robotic surgeons regarding long-term outcomes and appropriate patient selection.

The debate over the optimal minimally invasive approach continues to highlight another great issue of our time and that is the state of gynecologic surgical training. With fellowship directors reporting that less than 50% of recent graduates are able to independently perform a hysterectomy by any route,[46] more research must be completed on how to improve resident training in general before the introduction of additional minimally invasive surgical technologies and techniques.

SUPPLEMENTARY DATA

Supplementary data related to this article can be found at http://dx.doi.org/10.1016/j.ogc.2016.04.008.

REFERENCES

1. Faust R. Robotics in surgery: history, current and future applications. New York: Nova Science Publishers; 2007.

2. Visco A, Advincula A. Robotic gynecologic surgery. Obstet Gynecol 2008;112(6): 1369–84.

3. Advincula A, Wang K. Evolving role and current state of robotics in minimally invasive gynecologic surgery. J Minim Invasive Gynecol 2009;16(3):291–301.

4. Intuitive Surgical–Investors–Investor Relations Home. Investorintuitivesurgical.com. 2016. Available at: http://investor.intuitivesurgical.com/phoenix.zhtml?c=122359&p=irol-irhome. Accessed March 10, 2016.

5. Whiteman M, Hillis S, Jamieson D, et al. Inpatient hysterectomy surveillance in the United States, 2000-2004. Am J Obstet Gynecol 2008;198(1):34.e1–7.
6. Cohen S, Vitonis A, Einarsson J. Updated hysterectomy surveillance and factors associated with minimally invasive hysterectomy. JSLS 2014;18(3). http://dx.doi.org/10.4293/jsls.2014.00096.
7. Wright J, Herzog T, Tsui J, et al. Nationwide trends in the performance of inpatient hysterectomy in the United States. Obstet Gynecol 2013;122(2 Pt 1):233–41.
8. Committee opinion no. 628: robotic surgery in gynecology. Obstet Gynecol 2015; 125(3):760–7.
9. AAGL Advancing Minimally Invasive Gynecology Worldwide. AAGL position statement: robotic-assisted laparoscopic surgery in benign gynecology. J Minim Invasive Gynecol 2013;20(1):2–9.
10. Goto A, Takeuchi S, Sugimura K, et al. Usefulness of Gd-DTPA contrast-enhanced dynamic MRI and serum determination of LDH and its isozymes in the differential diagnosis of leiomyosarcoma from degenerated leiomyoma of the uterus. Int J Gynecol Cancer 2002;12(4):354–61.
11. ACOG Practice Bulletin No. 104. Antibiotic prophylaxis for gynecologic procedures. Obstet Gynecol 2009;113(5):1180–9.
12. Robotics in practice: New angles on safer positioning. Contemporary OB/GYN. 2016. Available at: http://contemporaryobgyn.modernmedicine.com/contemporary-obgyn/news/modernmedicine/modern-medicine-feature-articles/robotics-practice-new-angles. Accessed March 10, 2016.
13. Klauschie J, Wechter M, Jacob K, et al. Use of anti-skid material and patient-positioning to prevent patient shifting during robotic-assisted gynecologic procedures. J Minim Invasive Gynecol 2010;17(4):504–7.
14. Greenberg JA. The Pink Pad—Pigazzi Patient Positioning System™. Rev Obstet Gynecol 2013;6(2):97–8.
15. Ghomi A, Kramer C, Askari R, et al. Trendelenburg position in gynecologic robotic-assisted surgery. J Minim Invasive Gynecol 2012;19(4):485–9.
16. SGO Clinical Practice Statement: Salpingectomy for Ovarian Cancer Prevention. SGO. 2013. Available at: https://www.sgo.org/clinical-practice/guidelines/sgo-clinical-practice-statement-salpingectomy-for-ovarian-cancer-prevention/. Accessed March 10, 2016.
17. Farquhar C, Sadler L, Harvey S, et al. The association of hysterectomy and menopause: a prospective cohort study. BJOG 2005;112(7):956–62.
18. Baggish M, Karram M. Atlas of pelvic anatomy and gynecologic surgery.
19. Schiavone M, Herzog T, Ananth C, et al. Feasibility and economic impact of same-day discharge for women who undergo laparoscopic hysterectomy. Am J Obstet Gynecol 2012;207(5):382.e1–9.
20. Lee S, Calderon B, Gardner G, et al. The feasibility and safety of same-day discharge after robotic-assisted hysterectomy alone or with other procedures for benign and malignant indications. Gynecol Oncol 2014;133(3):552–5.
21. Kilic G, Moore G, Elbatanony A, et al. Comparison of perioperative outcomes of total laparoscopic and robotically assisted hysterectomy for benign pathology during introduction of a robotic program. Obstet Gynecol Int 2011;2011:683703.
22. Patzkowsky K, As-Sanie S, Smorgick N, et al. Perioperative outcomes of robotic versus laparoscopic hysterectomy for benign disease. JSLS 2013;17(1):100–6.
23. Wright K, Jonsdottir G, Jorgensen S, et al. Costs and outcomes of abdominal, vaginal, laparoscopic and robotic hysterectomies. JSLS 2012;16(4):519–24.
24. Orady M, Hrynewych A, Nawfal A, et al. Comparison of robotic-assisted hysterectomy to other minimally invasive approaches. JSLS 2012;16(4):542–8.

25. Payne T, Dauterive F. A comparison of total laparoscopic hysterectomy to robotically assisted hysterectomy: surgical outcomes in a community practice. J Minim Invasive Gynecol 2008;15(3):286–91.
26. Shashoua A, Gill D, Locher S. Robotic-assisted total laparoscopic hysterectomy versus conventional total laparoscopic hysterectomy. JSLS 2009;13(3):364–9.
27. Liu H, Lawrie T, Lu D, et al. Robot-assisted surgery in gynaecology. Cochrane Database Syst Rev 2014. http://dx.doi.org/10.1002/14651858.cd011422.
28. Albright B, Witte T, Tofte A, et al. Robotic versus laparoscopic hysterectomy for benign disease: a systematic review and meta-analysis of randomized trials. J Minim Invasive Gynecol 2016;23(1):18–27.
29. Lenihan J, Kovanda C, Seshadri-Kreaden U. What is the learning curve for robotic assisted gynecologic surgery? J Minim Invasive Gynecol 2008;15(5): 589–94.
30. Woelk J, Casiano E, Weaver A, et al. The learning curve of robotic hysterectomy. Obstet Gynecol 2013;121(1):87–95.
31. Bell M, Hunt S. 28: the first hundred da Vinci hysterectomies: analysis of the learning curve for a single surgeon. J Minim Invasive Gynecol 2007;14(6):S11–2.
32. Smorgick N, DeLancey J, Patzkowsky K, et al. Risk factors for postoperative urinary retention after laparoscopic and robotic hysterectomy for benign indications. Obstet Gynecol 2012;120(3):581–6.
33. Nick A, Lange J, Frumovitz M, et al. Rate of vaginal cuff separation following laparoscopic or robotic hysterectomy. Gynecol Oncol 2011;120(1):47–51.
34. Kho R, Akl M, Cornella J, et al. Incidence and characteristics of patients with vaginal cuff dehiscence after robotic procedures. Obstet Gynecol 2009;114(2 Pt 1):231–5.
35. Uccella S, Ghezzi F, Mariani A, et al. Vaginal cuff closure after minimally invasive hysterectomy: our experience and systematic review of the literature. Am J Obstet Gynecol 2011;205(2):119.e1–12.
36. Bolenz C, Gupta A, Hotze T, et al. Cost comparison of robotic, laparoscopic, and open radical prostatectomy for prostate cancer. Eur Urol 2010;57(3):453–8.
37. Pasic R, Rizzo J, Fang H, et al. Comparing robot-assisted with conventional laparoscopic hysterectomy: impact on cost and clinical outcomes. J Minim Invasive Gynecol 2010;17(6):730–8.
38. Venkat P, Chen L, Young-Lin N, et al. An economic analysis of robotic versus laparoscopic surgery for endometrial cancer: costs, charges and reimbursements to hospitals and professionals. Gynecol Oncol 2012;125(1):237–40.
39. Barnett J, Judd J, Wu J, et al. Cost comparison among robotic, laparoscopic, and open hysterectomy for endometrial cancer. Obstet Gynecol 2010;116(3):685–93.
40. Holtz D, Miroshnichenko G, Finnegan M, et al. Endometrial cancer surgery costs: robot vs laparoscopy. J Minim Invasive Gynecol 2010;17(4):500–3.
41. Wright J, Ananth C, Tergas A, et al. An economic analysis of robotically assisted hysterectomy. Obstet Gynecol 2014;123(5):1038–48.
42. Lonnerfors C, Reynisson P, Persson J. A randomized trial comparing vaginal and laparoscopic hysterectomy vs robot-assisted hysterectomy. J Minim Invasive Gynecol 2015;22(1):78–86.
43. Boggess J, Gehrig P, Cantrell L, et al. Perioperative outcomes of robotically assisted hysterectomy for benign cases with complex pathology. Obstet Gynecol 2009;114(3):585–93.
44. Lim P, Crane J, English E, et al. Multicenter analysis comparing robotic, open, laparoscopic, and vaginal hysterectomies performed by high-volume surgeons

for benign indications. Int J Gynaecol Obstet 2016. http://dx.doi.org/10.1016/j.ijgo.2015.11.010.

45. Landeen L, Bell M, Hubert H, et al. Clinical and cost comparisons for hysterectomy via abdominal, standard laparoscopic, vaginal and robot-assisted approaches. S D Med 2011;64(6):197–9.

46. Guntupalli S, Doo D, Guy M, et al. Preparedness of obstetrics and gynecology residents for fellowship training. Obstet Gynecol 2015;126(3):559–68.

Evidence Basis for Hysterectomy

Jenifer N. Byrnes, DO, Emanuel C. Trabuco, MD, MS*

KEYWORDS

- Hysterectomy • Cuff dehiscence • Robotic • Vaginal • Laparoscopic • Costs

KEY POINTS

- National hysterectomy utilization has steadily declined since the early 1990s after the introduction of uterine-preserving treatments for fibroids and bleeding.
- Available evidence suggests that vaginal hysterectomy is cheaper and safer compared with other approaches.
- Both laparoscopic and robotic hysterectomy are associated with increased rates of vaginal cuff dehiscence compared with vaginal hysterectomy.
- Robotic hysterectomy has been shown to be consistently more expensive than other modes of hysterectomy with no identifiable advantages.
- Widespread adoption of robotic hysterectomy utilization has had a negative impact on obstetrics and gynecology residency training.

INTRODUCTION

Although hysterectomy remains the most commonly performed gynecologic surgery, annual rates have steadily decreased from a peak of 681,234 in 2002 to 433,621 yearly procedures in 2010.[1] Although the reason for the trend is likely multifactorial, increased utilization of minimally invasive, uterine-preserving conservative treatments for leiomyoma and abnormal uterine bleeding are the likely main drivers for the decrease in hysterectomy (see the articles by Laughlin-Tommaso SK: Alternatives to Hysterectomy: Management of Uterine Fibroids, and Billow MR, El-Nashar SA: Management of Abnormal Uterine Bleeding with Emphasis on Alternatives to Hysterectomy, in this issue).

Vaginal hysterectomy has long been regarded as the gold standard operation for uterine removal, owing to its minimally invasive approach with low morbidity and cost. Laparoscopy, first introduced in gynecology in 1990s, has progressively evolved from laparoscopic-assisted vaginal hysterectomy to total laparoscopic

Department of Obstetrics and Gynecology, Mayo Clinic, 200 First Street Southwest, Rochester, MN 55905, USA
* Corresponding author.
E-mail address: trabuco.emanuel@mayo.edu

Obstet Gynecol Clin N Am 43 (2016) 495–515
http://dx.doi.org/10.1016/j.ogc.2016.04.009
0889-8545/16/$ – see front matter © 2016 Elsevier Inc. All rights reserved.

uterine removal (**Box 1**). Although this minimally invasive approach afforded considerable benefit compared with abdominal hysterectomy, it has not gained widespread utilization given the steep learning curve. Since its introduction in 2005, robotic-assisted surgery has been widely adopted owning to improved ergonomics and imaging, wristed instruments, easier suturing compared with traditional laparoscopy, and an aggressive marketing campaign to physicians and hospitals. In fact, the proportion of hysterectomy performed robotically has grown from less than 1% in 2007 to 36% of all procedures performed in 2010.[2] Unfortunately, increased robotic utilization has significantly curtailed both abdominal and vaginal hysterectomy. The goal of next section of the article is to compare the different modes of hysterectomy.

Box 1 lists definitions and abbreviations for the different modes of hysterectomy reviewed in this article.

Box 1
Types of Hysterectomy

- Total abdominal hysterectomy (TAH)

- Vaginal hysterectomy (VH) or Total vaginal hysterectomy (TVH)

- Laparoscopic-assisted vaginal hysterectomy (LAVH)
  - Laparoscopic assistance up to, but not including division of the uterine arteries

- Laparoscopic hysterectomy (LH)
  - Laparoscopic division of the uterine arteries with completion of the procedure vaginally

- Total laparoscopic hysterectomy (TLH)
  - Entire portion, including vaginal cuff closure, performed laparoscopically

- Laparoscopic subtotal hysterectomy (LSH)
  - Removal of the uterine fundus with preservation of the cervix through either morcellation or mini-laparotomy

- Robotic-assisted laparoscopic hysterectomy (RH)

USING THE EVIDENCE TO CHOOSE THE BEST APPROACH
Vaginal Hysterectomy Versus Total Abdominal Hysterectomy

Few randomized trials compare abdominal with vaginal hysterectomy. Available studies credit vaginal hysterectomy with quicker return to normal activities,[3–5] decreased operative time,[3,5–7] and improved satisfaction and quality of life[8] with similar rates of visceral injury and estimated blood loss.[9] In one study with shorter mean operative time for abdominal hysterectomy (68 minutes vs 81 minutes), the mean hospital length of stay was significantly longer (3.7 days vs 2.8 days) and mean postoperative recovery occurred later (28.1 days vs 21.3 days).[3]

Data from the 2015 Cochrane review supports shorter operative time (mean difference [95% CI]: −11.01 [−35.09,13.08]), faster return to activity (mean difference [95% CI]: −12.33 days, [−19.89 to −4.77 days], shorter hospital stay (mean difference [95% CI]: −1.07 days [−1.22, −0.92 days]), and higher satisfaction (OR 2.69 [0.50, 14.42]) with vaginal compared to abdominal hysterectomy.[10] There was no difference in intraoperative complications, but there was a trend toward fewer postoperative complications favoring vaginal hysterectomy.

Table 1 provides a summary of key randomized studies comparing vaginal with abdominal hysterectomy.

Vaginal Hysterectomy Versus Laparoscopic Hysterectomy

"Laparoscopic hysterectomy" may be used to refer to any one of several variations in technique,[11] making it more challenging to apply evidence widely. Munro and Parker[12] developed a classification system for laparoscopic hysterectomy to accurately track outcomes and complication rates. Most studies discussed in this article compared vaginal to laparoscopic assisted or total laparoscopic hysterectomy (see **Box 1**).

A Cochrane review found no benefit to laparoscopic-assisted vaginal hysterectomy over vaginal hysterectomy, with vaginal hysterectomy being associated with shorter operative time (mean difference [95% CI]: 33.69 [20.13–47.07]).[10] Similar findings were reported in a meta-analysis of 9 studies comparing laparoscopic-assisted vaginal hysterectomy with vaginal hysterectomy; women who had a vaginal hysterectomy had shorter operative time (mean difference [95% CI]: 39.59 min [20.00–59.18 min], $P<.001$) and trend toward shorter hospital stay (mean difference [95% CI]: 1.17 days [–0.1–2.43 days]; P .07) and fewer conversions (OR 2.21 [0.092–5.32]; $P = .08$).[13] There was no difference in complications, blood loss, ileus, or uterine weight between groups.

Vaginal hysterectomy also had shorter operative time compared with laparoscopic hysterectomy (mean difference [95% CI]: 53.58 min [43.67–63.49 min]) and total laparoscopic hysterectomy (mean difference [95% CI]: 17.3 min [3.34–31.26 min]).[10] There were no differences in intraoperative visceral injury or bleeding complications, conversion rates, or major short-term (hematoma, infection, or thromboembolic events) or long-term complications (fistula or urinary dysfunction). There were no differences in return to normal activities between laparoscopic (all subtypes) and vaginal hysterectomy groups. One study found higher patient satisfaction with vaginal hysterectomy and total laparoscopic hysterectomy compared with laparoscopic-assisted vaginal hysterectomy at the 6-month follow-up visit ($P = .003$).[14]

Table 2 summarizes the findings of studies comparing vaginal with laparoscopic hysterectomy.

Vaginal Hysterectomy Versus Robotic Hysterectomy

There are no randomized trials comparing vaginal and robotic hysterectomy. Available data indicate robotic hysterectomy has no significant advantage over conventional laparoscopic hysterectomy[24] and is associated with higher cost even after adjusting for surgeon volume (**Box 2**).[25] Longer surgical times associated with robotic surgery have been linked to increased postoperative pulmonary complications, possibly related to increased time spent in Trendelenburg position.[24]

In a recent large retrospective cohort study, Woelk and colleagues[26] compared these approaches using 1-to-1 propensity score matching to ensure similar baseline characteristics and minimize the risk of selection bias inherent in cohort study design. Robotic surgery was associated with higher postoperative complication rates (15.1% vs 8.0%; $P = .02$) and longer operative time (1.2 vs 0.7 hours; $P \leq .001$) but shorter hospitalization (1 vs 2 mean days; $P \leq .001$) and higher mean uterine weight (243.4 ± 300.1 vs 165.3 ± 151.8; $P \leq .001$). There was no difference in intraoperative complications between groups.

COST DIFFERENCES

There is an increasing body of literature regarding cost trends in gynecologic surgery, but cost measures have been inconsistent. This is particularly problematic with robotic hysterectomy, as reported costs frequently fail to include purchase price or annual maintenance of the robot. Robotic surgical systems are reported to have a fixed initial

Table 1
Summary of selected prospective randomized studies comparing vaginal hysterectomy with abdominal hysterectomy

Study (Country), Year, Design	Uterine Weight	Operative Time	Estimated Blood Loss	Intraoperative Complications	Hospital LOS	Pain Control	Postoperative Complications	Return to Activity	QOL/ Satisfaction	Discussion and Conclusions
				Main Variables Evaluated						
Ribeiro et al (Brazil),[6] 2003, n = 60	X	X	X	X	—	—	X	—	—	• All cases performed by 1 surgeon • Mean uterine weight: TAH 189.5 g, VH 155.65 g, LH 154.5 g • VH is superior to both TAH and LH in operative time and inflammatory response measured by serum markers ○ Mean operative time (min): TAH 109, VH 78, LH 119 (P .001)
Hwang et al (Taiwan),[5] 2002, n = 90	X	X	X	—	X	X	X	X	—	• Cases performed by 1 author with 2 author assistance • Larger mean uterine weight in TAH group (1020 g) than TVH (835 g) and LAVH (748 g) groups. (P 0.02) • VH: shortest operative time, lowest blood loss, shortest hospital stay, lowest risk of infection, fastest bowel recovery and lowest pain score (vs LH and TAH) • Severe pelvic adhesions from endometriosis and uterine fibroids >13 cm were the only CI to VH or LH

Study							Comments
Ottosen et al (Sweden),[3] 2000, n = 120	X	X	X	X	—	X	—	• Cases performed by 15 surgeons and supervised residents • LH significantly longer operative time (102 min vs 68 min TAH and 81 VH min) • TAH significantly longer hospital LOS (2.7 d vs 2.8 d VH and 3.1 d LH) • TAH significantly longer time to recovery (28.1 d vs 21.3 d VH and 19.7 d LH) • Authors recommend using laparoscopy to judge accessibility of the uterus, rule out presence of adhesive disease, then turn to the vaginal portion
Benassi et al (Italy),[7] 2002, n = 119	X	X	X	X	X	—	X	• Cases performed by experienced GYN surgeons (no quantification reported) • No difference in mean uterine weight 380 g vs 436 g (AH) • Operative time significantly longer for TAH (102 min) vs VH (86 min) • Significantly longer hospital LOS for AH (4.2 d) vs VH (3.4 d) • Cost significantly higher for AH vs VH • Enlarged uterus does not preclude vaginal hysterectomy

Abbreviations: AH, abdominal hysterectomy; CI, contraindications; GYN, gynecology; LAVH, laparoscopic-assisted vaginal hysterectomy; LH, laparoscopic hysterectomy; LOS, length of stay; QOL, quality of life; TAH, total abdominal hysterectomy; TVH, total vaginal hysterectomy; VH, vaginal hysterectomy.

Table 2
Summary of selected prospective randomized studies comparing vaginal hysterectomy with laparoscopic hysterectomy

Study (Country), Year, Design	Uterine Weight	Operative Time	Blood Loss	Intraoperative Complications	Hospital LOS	Pain Control	Postoperative Complications	Return to Activity	QOL/ Satisfaction	Discussion and Conclusions
					Main Variables Evaluated					
Ghezzi et al (Italy),[15] 2010, n = 82	X	X	X	X	X	—	X	X	—	• Patients in LH group experienced significantly less pain, as measured by VAS score at various time intervals, and number of patients requesting a 10-mg SQ dose of morphine analgesic, than VH group • LH independent predictor for shorter LOS • No conversions to laparotomy, intraoperative complications, or blood transfusion in either group.
Drahonovsky et al (Czech Republic),[16] 2010, n = 125	X	X	X	X	X	X	X	—	—	• Operative time significantly shorter for VH (66 min [30–166 min]) vs LAVH (85 min [40–150 min]) and LH (111 min [55–180 min]). • Mean blood loss highest for LAVH (306 mL [35–1300 mL]) vs VH (208 mL [30–670 mL]) and LH (184 mL [14–700 mL])

| Sesti et al (Italy),[17] 2008, n = 80 | X | X | X | — | X | X | — | — |

- Analgesic consumption (units of 50 mg tramadol) lowest for LAVH (3.4) and highest for VH (4.8)
- Although conversion rate did not differ significantly, the 3 VH procedures were converted to LAVH due to complications during salpingo-oophorectomy
- Cases performed by 2 surgeons
- Vaginal hysterectomy had significantly lower operative time (VH 71 ± 3 min vs LH 129 ± 7 min), estimated blood loss (VH 186.0 mL ± 52 vs LH 362.7 ± 65 mL), and time to hospital discharge (VH 48 ± 2.6 h vs LH 72 ± 4.2 h), and postoperative ileus (VH: 19 ± 3 h vs LH: 26 ± 3 h)
- LH was associated with more postoperative pain and fever.
- No intraoperative complications, conversion to laparotomy, or major postoperative complications in either group.

(continued on next page)

Table 2
(continued)

Study (Country), Year, Design	Uterine Weight	Operative Time	Blood Loss	Intraoperative Complications	Hospital LOS	Pain Control	Postoperative Complications	Return to Activity	QOL/ Satisfaction	Discussion and Conclusions
				Main Variables Evaluated						
Agostini et al (France),[18] 2006, n = 48	X	X	X	X	X	—	X	—	—	• Cases performed by 5 senior surgeons • No difference in operative time (VH 83.9 ± 34.6 min vs LH 100.2 ± 27.9 min) or hospital stay (VH 5.5 d vs LH 5.6 d). • Overall complication rate significantly higher for LH (54.1%) vs VH (25%), which included estimated blood loss, trocar port hematoma, vaginal cuff hematoma, and postoperative fever.
Garry et al (South Africa),[19] 2004, n = 1346	X	X	X	X	X	X	X	—	X	• 2 Concurrent RCT: LH vs TAH, LH vs VH. • Approach to LH not standardized. • No difference in pain scores for VH vs LH. • All procedures associated with improved quality of life on SF-12 score, body image scale, and aspects of sexual activity. ○ 937 followed-up at 1 y.

						• Operative time significantly shorter for VH (46.6 min [14–168 min]) vs LH (76.5 min [21–220 min]). • VH vs LH underpowered to detect significant differences other than operative time.
Ribeiro et al (Brazil),[6] 2003, n = 60	X	X	X	X	—	—	• All cases performed by 1 surgeon. • Mean uterine weight: TAH 189.5 g, VH 155.65 g, LH 154.5 g. • VH is superior to both TAH and LH in operative time and inflammatory response measured by serum markers. ○ Mean operative time (min): TAH 109, VH 78, LH 119 (*P* .001).

(continued on next page)

Table 2
(continued)

Study (Country), Year, Design	Uterine Weight	Operative Time	Blood Loss	Intraoperative Complications	Hospital LOS	Pain Control	Postoperative Complications	Return to Activity	QOL/ Satisfaction	Discussion and Conclusions
				Main Variables Evaluated						
Hwang et al (Taiwan),[5] 2002, n = 90	X	X	X	—	X	X	X	X	—	• Cases performed by 1 author with 2 author assistance. • Larger mean uterine weight in TAH group (1020 g) than TVH (835 g) and LAVH (748 g) groups (*P* .02). • VH: shortest operative time, lowest blood loss, shortest hospital stay, lowest risk of infection, fastest bowel recovery and lowest pain score (vs LH and TAH). • Severe pelvic adhesions from endometriosis and uterine fibroids >13 cm were the only CI to VH or LH.
Daraï et al, (France),[20] 2001, n = 80	X	X	X	X	X	—	X	—	—	• Included women with uterine weight >280 g. • Experienced surgeons (no quantification). • In the VH group, there were 13 cases (32.5%) of uterine size at least 500 g

and 4 cases of uterine size at least 700 g, in which all the operations were completed vaginally.
- Significantly higher rate of conversion to laparotomy higher for LH (7.5%) vs VH (0%).
- Significantly higher minor (15% VH vs 37.5% LH) and major (2.5 VH vs 12.5% LH) complications in LH.

Soriano et al (France),[21] 2001, n = 80

- Mean uterine weight similar between groups (VH: 424 ± 211 g vs LH: 481 ± 329 g)
- Vaginal hysterectomy had significantly shorter operative time (VH 108 ± 35 min vs LH 160 ± 50 min) and lower complication rate (VH 15% vs LH 32.5%).
- No difference in change in hemoglobin, consumption of pain medication (after excluding 3 women requiring laparotomy in LH group), or time to flatus/BM.

(continued on next page)

Table 2
(continued)

Study (Country), Year, Design	Uterine Weight	Operative Time	Blood Loss	Intraoperative Complications	Hospital LOS	Pain Control	Postoperative Complications	Return to Activity	QOL/ Satisfaction	Discussion and Conclusions
					Main Variables Evaluated					
Ottosen et al (Sweden),[3] 2000, n = 120	X	X	X	X	X	—	—	X	—	• Cases performed by 15 surgeons and supervised residents. • LH significantly longer operative time (102 min vs 68 min TAH and 81 min VH min). • TAH significantly longer hospital LOS (2.7 d vs 2.8 d VH and 3.1 d LH). • TAH significantly longer recovery time (28.1 d vs 21.3 d VH and 19.7 d LH). • Authors recommend using laparoscopy to judge accessibility of the uterus, rule out presence of adhesive disease, then turn to the vaginal portion.
Richardson et al (England),[22] 1995, n = 98	X	X	X	X	X	X	X	X	—	• Study began after a "learning curve" period for surgeons involved. • Surgery was completed with the intended technique in 93.9% of cases. 5 women in the LH group (6.7%) and 2 in the VH

Study										Notes
Summitt et al (USA),[23] 1992, n = 56	X	X	X	X	X	X	—	—	—	• Cases performed by an operating team of 3 surgeons: 2 attending faculty and 1 senior resident. • Women undergoing LAVH had statistically more prior surgeries than VH (1.42 vs 0.82). • Operative time was significantly longer for LH (120.1 ± 28.5 min) vs VH (64.7 ± 27 min). • Estimated blood loss was significantly higher for VH (376.1 ± 261.5 mL) vs LH (203.8 ± 130.5 mL). • Adnexectomy able to be performed 100% in both groups when indicated. • Cost was significantly higher for LH ($7904) vs VH ($4891). • LAVH had lower hematocrit readings 24 and 48 h after surgery. • group required laparotomy or additional procedures. • No *P* values reported.

Abbreviations: BM, bowel movement; LAVH, laparoscopic-assisted vaginal hysterectomy; LH, laparoscopic hysterectomy; LOS, length of stay; QOL, quality of life; RCT, randomized controlled trial; SQ, subcutaneous; TAH, total abdominal hysterectomy; VAS, visual analog scale; VH, vaginal hysterectomy.

Box 2
Summary of findings from comparative studies between modes of hysterectomy

Vaginal Hysterectomy versus Total Abdominal Hysterectomy

- Quicker return to normal activity
- Decreased operative time
- Decreased cost
- Improved patient satisfaction, cosmesis and quality of life

Vaginal Hysterectomy versus Laparoscopic Hysterectomy

- Shorter operative time
- Decreased cost

Vaginal Hysterectomy versus Robotic Hysterectomy

- Decreased cost
- No level I evidence

Data from Refs.[24,34–36]

---

purchase cost up to $2.5 million and an annual maintenance contract priced at 10% of the cost of the unit.[27] Disposable proprietary wristed instruments can be used only 10 times each and cost $2000 to $3000 per instrument.

Beyond the cost of the robotic system, surgeons and hospitals lose productivity due to longer operative time. These "opportunity costs" can be difficult to measure, but contribute significantly to the disparity between cost of robotic and vaginal approaches. In a study using simulated data based on surgical time and hospital revenue, 16 fewer hysterectomies could be performed each month if the robot was used for cases that were previously performed laparoscopically.[28] This translated to an annual loss of $1.9 to $2.5 million. The 2013 position statement released by the American Association of Gynecologic Laparoscopists estimated that the health care system would incur an additional $960 million to $1.9 billion in cost if each of the 600,000 annual hysterectomies performed in the United States were completed robotically.[27]

In a retrospective study using data extracted from Allscripts, Dayaratna and colleagues[29] found vaginal hysterectomy to be the only approach that generated income when evaluating hospital cost and net revenue for vaginal, laparoscopic-assisted vaginal hysterectomy, total laparoscopic hysterectomy, and robotic hysterectomies. In this study, the mean income generated from vaginal hysterectomy was $1200 per procedure, whereas total laparoscopic hysterectomy and robotic hysterectomies were associated with losses of $4000 per procedure. The investigators performed a secondary analysis in 149 cases that were treated laparoscopically or robotically but which could have been treated by a vaginal approach. Subjects were selected using intentionally conservative criteria, including a history of at least 1 prior vaginal delivery, less than 1 previous laparotomy, and a uterine size less than 14 weeks' gestation. Of the 149 nonvaginal cases, 64 laparoscopic-assisted vaginal hysterectomy, 6 total laparoscopic hysterectomy, and 13 robotic hysterectomies met the conservative criteria and could have been performed vaginally. The investigators estimated that the hospital could have saved $273,720, not including the purchase and maintenance cost for the robot, if they have performed these procedures by the vaginal route. As in other studies, operative time was significantly longer for robotic and laparoscopic approaches.[3,5,6,16,17,21,28]

Woelk and colleagues[26] used the Olmsted County Healthcare Expenditure and Utilization Database to compare all-cause costs through the first 6 postoperative weeks between robotic and vaginal hysterectomy. Despite not accounting for robot acquisition, maintenance, and instrument costs, robotic hysterectomy cost an average of $2253 (95% CI $972–$3535) more than vaginal hysterectomy. This cost persisted in the subgroups that did not experience a postoperative or intraoperative complication (mean $2154). Hospital costs were significantly greater in women who had an intraoperative ($6016) or postoperative complication ($5020) compared with those without a complication, but there was no difference between vaginal and robotic subgroups experiencing either of the complications.

It appears that the unit cost of robotic hysterectomy far exceeds the unit cost of vaginal hysterectomy with no demonstrable improvement in outcomes[30] and questions the cost-benefit equation concerning the widespread adaptation of robotic hysterectomy.

VAGINAL CUFF DEHISCENCE

Although the rate of vaginal cuff dehiscence varies drastically by mode of hysterectomy,[31–34] this rare, but morbid and costly complication is seldom included in meta-analyses and Cochrane reviews. Patients experiencing this complication commonly present with bloody vaginal discharge or report a sudden gush of fluid per vagina, typically following coitus.[31,32] Treatment requires universal return to the operating room with up to 29% requiring bowel resection due to evisceration-related small bowel ischemia.[32]

Dehiscence rates following vaginal hysterectomy are low, ranging from 0.032% to 0.13%.[34,35] Patients experiencing this complication present at a median follow-up of 2 years after hysterectomy. Conversely, cuff dehiscence rates following total laparoscopic hysterectomy range from 0.64% to 4.9%[32,36] and present at a median of 1 to 3 months after surgery.[32,36] Hur and colleagues[36] reported dehiscence rates in a series of 7039 women undergoing hysterectomy at Magee-Womens Hospital between January 2000 and March 2006. Although the overall dehiscence rate was 0.24%, and similar to other publications, the dehiscence rates following laparoscopic hysterectomy was higher compared with vaginal and abdominal approaches and reached 4.93% for the January 2005 to March 2006 time frame.

Recently, the investigators updated their incidence data by collecting dehiscence rates between January 2006 and December 2009.[33] Although the 10-year cumulative incidence of cuff dehiscence following total laparoscopic hysterectomy decreased from the previously reported 4.93% to 1.35%, cuff dehiscence rates remained significantly higher following total laparoscopic hysterectomy compared with vaginal hysterectomy (1.35% vs 0.08%; $P<.001$). The risk ratio for cuff dehiscence was 17.2-fold higher following laparoscopic compared with vaginal hysterectomy (95% CI 3.5–75.9).

Another series of 12,398 women undergoing hysterectomy at 6 Italian hospitals between January 1994 and December 2008 reported increased rates of vaginal cuff dehiscence following laparoscopic compared with vaginal hysterectomy (0.64% vs 0.13%); with the former being associated with a 4.9-fold increased risk of dehiscence ($P<.001$; OR 4.9, 95% CI 2.00–12.06). Interestingly, there was no difference in the risk of dehiscence in the subgroup of women who underwent laparoscopy hysterectomy with vaginal closure compared with women who had a vaginal hysterectomy (0.24% vs 0.13%; $P = .39$, OR 1.15. 95% CI 0.46–7.33). This finding would suggest that surgical technique rather than thermal damage incurred during laparoscopic colpotomy may account for most of the increased risk of dehiscence following laparoscopic hysterectomy.[37]

Although less well studied, robotic hysterectomy is also associated with increased risk of cuff dehiscence, with rates ranging from 3.0% to 4.1%.[31,38] It is concerning that the rates of dehiscence increased form 1.5% in 2005 to 6.8% in 2008, because one would expect decreased complications with progression through the learning curve.[31] The authors, and others, have hypothesized that the increased rates were due to thermal damage associated with monopolar coagulation current (50 W) during colpotomy, but there are no data that altering the current type and strength mitigates this complication.

ADDITIONAL FACTORS TO CONSIDER
Increasing Vaginal Hysterectomy Utilization

Even though there are a number of widely reported "contraindications" to vaginal hysterectomy (eg, nulliparity, narrow pubic arch or vagina, history of laparotomy including cesarean delivery, absence of uterine descensus, or significant uterine enlargement), there is a wide body of evidence that vaginal hysterectomy can be safely performed in more than 90% of the cases with these risk factors.

Several studies have shown vaginal hysterectomy can be successfully completed in the presence of enlarged uteri.[5,7,20,21] A randomized trial comparing vaginal and abdominal approaches in a population of women with enlarged uteri (mean uterine weight 380 ± 165 g) reported no difference in intraoperative complications between groups.[7] In a prospective trial of 300 women undergoing vaginal hysterectomy for non-prolapsed uteri, including nulliparous women and those with previous pelvic surgery, 99% of cases were completed vaginally, with 1% intraoperative complication rate.[39] All 3 failures occurred following hysterectomy due to inability to complete adnexectomy vaginally. In a case-control study of 5092 women undergoing hysterectomy at 3 Cincinnati hospitals, there was an overall increased risk of bladder injury during hysterectomy in patients with a history of cesarean delivery (OR 2.04, 95% CI 1.2–3.5; $P = .005$); however, when the hysterectomy subgroups were analyzed (total abdominal hysterectomy, vaginal hysterectomy, and laparoscopic-assisted vaginal hysterectomy) only the laparoscopic-assisted group had a statistically significant increased risk of bladder injury (OR 7.50, 95% CI 1.8–31.4: $P = .005$). A smaller retrospective study similarly found no difference in complication rates in women undergoing vaginal hysterectomy with or without a history of cesarean delivery (11.3% vs 4.3%, respectively; $P = .10$).[40]

Despite the overwhelming evidence presented regarding the safety and success of vaginal hysterectomy in patients with these relative "contraindications," the continued national decline in vaginal hysterectomy begs the question of whether it is possible to improve vaginal hysterectomy utilization. Kovac and colleagues[41] compared vaginal hysterectomy rates before and after implementation of simple guidelines (vagina is >2 finger breadths at the apex or the cervix is stage 1 or higher on examination) to identify potential candidates for vaginal hysterectomy for benign indications in a residency-training program. Patients who had limited descensus or enlarged uteri underwent examination under anesthesia, and those who had historical factors suspicious for extrauterine disease (endometriosis, pelvic inflammatory disease, ovarian pathology, or chronic pelvic pain) underwent diagnostic laparoscopy with a 5-mm scope. If no disease was detected, the remainder of the procedure was completed vaginally without laparoscopic assistance. By implementing these simple guidelines, the investigators succeeded in changing the abdominal to vaginal hysterectomy ratios from 3:1 to 1:11; with vaginal hysterectomy accomplished in 91.8% of the cases (374 of 407).[41] Uterine size reduction techniques were successful in 82.2% (37/45) of the women with estimated uterine weight greater than 280 g. Moreover, diagnostic laparoscopy revealed absent or mild extrauterine pathology in 90.9% (80/88) of the patients with the previously mentioned historical risk factors for extrauterine disease; allowing for completion of vaginal hysterectomy without any additional laparoscopic assistance.

This study demonstrated that adoption of simple guidelines in a residency program could safely increase vaginal hysterectomy utilization. Patients with enlarged uteri or who lacked descensus needed only undergo an examination under anesthesia to assess for vaginal access. Patients with historical risk factors suggestive of adhesive disease lacked significant disease, precluding vaginal hysterectomy 90% of the time. Diagnostic laparoscopy to screen these patients with a 5-mm scope did not add significantly to the operative time. This study clearly demonstrated the ease and safety of identifying eligible patients for vaginal surgeries that could readily be applied to other clinical settings.

Increased Risk of Prolapse

The conflicting evidence regarding mode of hysterectomy and risk of future prolapse repair has served to perpetuate the widespread misconception that hysterectomy predisposes to prolapse.[42–44] A large population-based Swedish study comparing rates of subsequent prolapse repair among women undergoing hysterectomy (n = 162,488) and controls (n = 470,519) with intact reproductive tracts, demonstrated that all modes of hysterectomy were associated with increased risk of prolapse repair.[43] Specifically, women older than 55 years at the time of hysterectomy and those who had a vaginal procedure had the highest risk. Although large and based on a robust nationwide database, this study was limited by the small proportion of participants undergoing a vaginal hysterectomy (only 6%) and more importantly, for failure to adjust for the presence or absence of baseline pelvic organ prolapse.[43]

Two robustly designed studies have addressed this question while adjusting for the presence or absence of baseline pelvic organ prolapse. The first was a population-based cohort study evaluating the incidence of pelvic floor repairs among Olmsted County women who had hysterectomy with and without combined prolapse repairs between 1965 and 2002. Unlike the previously mentioned study, the cumulative incidence of needing pelvic floor repairs was low and similar between vaginal and abdominal hysterectomy groups at 20 years (2.1% [95% CI 1.3–2.8] versus 1.9 [95% CI 1.0–2.8]; $P = .41$) if patients had no pelvic organ prolapse at baseline (eg, had a hysterectomy for fibroids or bleeding). However, the incidence of reoperation increased to 9.5% (95% CI 5.1–14.6) among women who had baseline prolapse and underwent isolated vaginal hysterectomy. If women with baseline prolapse had concomitant repairs at the time of the index hysterectomy, the incidence of reoperation for prolapse decreased to 4.4% (95% CI 3.4–5.4). Similar findings were observed for the subgroups of women undergoing abdominal hysterectomy.[42] A case-control study of women undergoing hysterectomy for benign indications at Geneva University Hospital between 1982 and 2002 has yielded similar results. Whereas the overall incidence of needing subsequent prolapse repairs for all women in the cohort was only 2.3%, the incidence of reoperation in the subgroup of women in baseline grade 2 or greater prolapse increased to approximately 7.5% at 23-year follow-up. Interestingly, the risk of reoperation was higher among women with grade 2 or greater prolapse regardless of the specifically impacted vaginal compartment (OR of future repairs 6.6 [95% CI

3.6–12.2], 5.2 [95% CI 2.7–10.0], 4.9 [95% CI 2.0–12.0]), if participants had anterior, posterior, or apical prolapse of 2 or greater compared with no prolapse, respectively ($P \leq .001$ for all comparisons). Multivariate logistic regression showed preoperative prolapse grade 2 or greater was the most important risk factor predicting the need for future repairs; increasing the risk of reoperation 12.6-fold ($P < .001$). Vaginal hysterectomy was not associated with increased risk of pelvic floor repairs after adjusting for confounders.[44] These data suggest that the degree of baseline prolapse, not the mode of hysterectomy, is the key determinant of whether or not a woman undergoing hysterectomy will require future prolapse repairs. Moreover, women undergoing vaginal hysterectomy incur no additional risk of developing prolapse; with a low, 1.9% cumulative incidence of undergoing another operation at 20 years' follow-up if she had no prolapse at the time of the index hysterectomy.

Impact on Trainees

The decrease in national vaginal hysterectomy utilization following the introduction of robotic hysterectomy has had a negative impact on resident education, with the number of vaginal hysterectomies performed by graduating trainees declining over the past decade.[45] Survey studies evaluating the proportion of newly graduating residents reporting being able to independently perform vaginal hysterectomy independently has markedly decreased from 79% in 2007 to 27.8% in 2010. More than 74% of residents cited that the robot has had a negative impact on surgical training. These studies highlight the need to increase trainee exposure to vaginal hysterectomy during residency. Surgeons who do not acquire these skills during training will likely fail to acquire them after graduation given the paucity of resources for further vaginal surgical skills training and competition from companies promoting and supporting laparoscopic and robotic surgery.

SUMMARY

Hysterectomy utilization has steadily declined over the past decade, whereas the number of approaches to hysterectomy has increased. The widespread adoption of robotic hysterectomy has not only eroded the proportion of abdominal but also vaginal hysterectomies. Unfortunately, the data reviewed in this article do not support this shift, as vaginal hysterectomy is quicker, cheaper, and associated with fewer complications compared with other approaches, including robotic hysterectomy. Robotic and laparoscopic hysterectomies are associated with significantly higher rates of cuff dehiscence; a rare but morbid complication that necessitates universal return to the operating room.

When guidelines are implemented to screen eligible patients (examination under anesthesia and diagnostic laparoscopy in patients with historical risk factors for adhesive disease), commonly cited contraindications do not appear to be an obstacle to the safe performance of vaginal hysterectomy. Prolapse following hysterectomy appears to be unrelated to the mode of hysterectomy, but rather whether or not a woman has stage 2 or greater prolapse at baseline. The changing trends in hysterectomy utilization are having a negative impact on resident education, with fewer than 30% reporting being able to independently perform vaginal hysterectomy in 2010. Realigning these trends may prove essential to continue to train residents in vaginal surgical skills and to allow our specialty to provide safe and cost-effective patient care.

REFERENCES

1. Wright JD, Herzog TJ, Tsui J, et al. Nationwide trends in the performance of inpatient hysterectomy in the United States. Obstet Gynecol 2013;122(2 Pt 1):233–41.
2. Pitter MC, Simmonds C, Seshadri-Kreaden U, et al. The impact of different surgical modalities for hysterectomy on satisfaction and patient reported outcomes. Interact J Med Res 2014;3(3):e11.
3. Ottosen C, Lingman G, Ottosen L. Three methods for hysterectomy: a randomised, prospective study of short term outcome. BJOG 2000;107(11):1380–5.
4. Miskry T, Magos A. Randomized, prospective, double-blind comparison of abdominal and vaginal hysterectomy in women without uterovaginal prolapse. Acta Obstet Gynecol Scand 2003;82(4):351–8.
5. Hwang JL, Seow KM, Tsai YL, et al. Comparative study of vaginal, laparoscopically assisted vaginal and abdominal hysterectomies for uterine myoma larger than 6 cm in diameter or uterus weighing at least 450 g: a prospective randomized study. Acta Obstet Gynecol Scand 2002;81(12):1132–8.
6. Ribeiro SC, Ribeiro RM, Santos NC, et al. A randomized study of total abdominal, vaginal and laparoscopic hysterectomy. Int J Gynaecol Obstet 2003;83(1):37–43.
7. Benassi L, Rossi T, Kaihura CT, et al. Abdominal or vaginal hysterectomy for enlarged uteri: a randomized clinical trial. Am J Obstet Gynecol 2002;187(6):1561–5.
8. Silva-Filho AL, Werneck RA, de Magalhães RS, et al. Abdominal vs vaginal hysterectomy: a comparative study of the postoperative quality of life and satisfaction. Arch Gynecol Obstet 2006;274(1):21–4.
9. Nieboer TE, Johnson N, Lethaby A, et al. Surgical approach to hysterectomy for benign gynaecological disease. Cochrane Database Syst Rev 2009;(3): CD003677.
10. Aarts JW, Nieboer TE, Johnson N, et al. Surgical approach to hysterectomy for benign gynaecological disease. Cochrane Database Syst Rev 2015;(8): CD003677.
11. Leung SW, Chan CS, Lo SF, et al. Comparison of the different types of "laparoscopic total hysterectomy". J Minim Invasive Gynecol 2007;14(1):91–6.
12. Munro MG, Parker WH. A classification system for laparoscopic hysterectomy. Obstet Gynecol 1993;82(4 Pt 1):624–9.
13. Guo Y, Tian X, Wang L. Laparoscopically assisted vaginal hysterectomy vs vaginal hysterectomy: meta-analysis. J Minim Invasive Gynecol 2013;20(1):15–21.
14. Roy KK, Goyal M, Singla S, et al. A prospective randomised study of total laparoscopic hysterectomy, laparoscopically assisted vaginal hysterectomy and nondescent vaginal hysterectomy for the treatment of benign diseases of the uterus. Arch Gynecol Obstet 2011;284(4):907–12.
15. Ghezzi F, Uccella S, Cromi A, et al. Postoperative pain after laparoscopic and vaginal hysterectomy for benign gynecologic disease: a randomized trial. Am J Obstet Gynecol 2010;203(2):118.e1–8.
16. Drahonovsky J, Haakova L, Otcenasek M, et al. A prospective randomized comparison of vaginal hysterectomy, laparoscopically assisted vaginal hysterectomy, and total laparoscopic hysterectomy in women with benign uterine disease. Eur J Obstet Gynecol Reprod Biol 2010;148(2):172–6.
17. Sesti F, Calonzi F, Ruggeri V, et al. A comparison of vaginal, laparoscopic-assisted vaginal, and minilaparotomy hysterectomies for enlarged myomatous uteri. Int J Gynaecol Obstet 2008;103(3):227–31.

18. Agostini A, Vejux N, Bretelle F, et al. Value of laparoscopic assistance for vaginal hysterectomy with prophylactic bilateral oophorectomy. Am J Obstet Gynecol 2006;194(2):351–4.

19. Garry R, Fountain J, Mason S, et al. The eVALuate study: two parallel randomised trials, one comparing laparoscopic with abdominal hysterectomy, the other comparing laparoscopic with vaginal hysterectomy. BMJ 2004;328(7432):129.

20. Daraï E, Soriano D, Kimata P, et al. Vaginal hysterectomy for enlarged uteri, with or without laparoscopic assistance: randomized study. Obstet Gynecol 2001; 97(5 Pt 1):712–6.

21. Soriano D, Goldstein A, Lecuru F, et al. Recovery from vaginal hysterectomy compared with laparoscopy-assisted vaginal hysterectomy: a prospective, randomized, multicenter study. Acta Obstet Gynecol Scand 2001;80(4):337–41.

22. Richardson RE, Bournas N, Magos AL. Is laparoscopic hysterectomy a waste of time? Lancet 1995;345(8941):36–41.

23. Summitt RL, Stovall TG, Lipscomb GH, et al. Randomized comparison of laparoscopy-assisted vaginal hysterectomy with standard vaginal hysterectomy in an outpatient setting. Obstet Gynecol 1992;80(6):895–901.

24. Rosero EB, Kho KA, Joshi GP, et al. Comparison of robotic and laparoscopic hysterectomy for benign gynecologic disease. Obstet Gynecol 2013;122(4):778–86.

25. Wright JD, Ananth CV, Tergas AI, et al. An economic analysis of robotically assisted hysterectomy. Obstet Gynecol 2014;123(5):1038–48.

26. Woelk JL, Borah BJ, Trabuco EC, et al. Cost differences among robotic, vaginal, and abdominal hysterectomy. Obstet Gynecol 2014;123(2 Pt 1):255–62.

27. AAGL Advancing Minimally Invasive Gynecology Worldwide. AAGL position statement: Robotic-assisted laparoscopic surgery in benign gynecology. J Minim Invasive Gynecol 2013;20(1):2–9.

28. Tiwari V. Calculating the true cost of robotic hysterectomy. Healthc Financ Manage 2014;68(8):80–5.

29. Dayaratna S, Goldberg J, Harrington C, et al. Hospital costs of total vaginal hysterectomy compared with other minimally invasive hysterectomy. Am J Obstet Gynecol 2014;210(2):120.e1–6.

30. Martino MA, Berger EA, McFetridge JT, et al. A comparison of quality outcome measures in patients having a hysterectomy for benign disease: robotic vs. non-robotic approaches. J Minim Invasive Gynecol 2014;21(3):389–93.

31. Kho RM, Akl MN, Cornella JL, et al. Incidence and characteristics of patients with vaginal cuff dehiscence after robotic procedures. Obstet Gynecol 2009;114(2 Pt 1):231–5.

32. Uccella S, Ceccaroni M, Cromi A, et al. Vaginal cuff dehiscence in a series of 12,398 hysterectomies: effect of different types of colpotomy and vaginal closure. Obstet Gynecol 2012;120(3):516–23.

33. Hur HC, Donnellan N, Mansuria S, et al. Vaginal cuff dehiscence after different modes of hysterectomy. Obstet Gynecol 2011;118(4):794–801.

34. Iaco PD, Ceccaroni M, Alboni C, et al. Transvaginal evisceration after hysterectomy: is vaginal cuff closure associated with a reduced risk? Eur J Obstet Gynecol Reprod Biol 2006;125(1):134–8.

35. Croak AJ, Gebhart JB, Klingele CJ, et al. Characteristics of patients with vaginal rupture and evisceration. Obstet Gynecol 2004;103(3):572–6.

36. Hur HC, Guido RS, Mansuria SM, et al. Incidence and patient characteristics of vaginal cuff dehiscence after different modes of hysterectomies. J Minim Invasive Gynecol 2007;14(3):311–7.

37. Uccella S, Ghezzi F, Mariani A, et al. Vaginal cuff closure after minimally invasive hysterectomy: our experience and systematic review of the literature. Am J Obstet Gynecol 2011;205(2):119.e1–12.
38. Nick AM, Lange J, Frumovitz M, et al. Rate of vaginal cuff separation following laparoscopic or robotic hysterectomy. Gynecol Oncol 2011;120(1):47–51.
39. Figueiredo O, Figueiredo EG, Figueiredo PG, et al. Vaginal removal of the benign nonprolapsed uterus: experience with 300 consecutive operations. Obstet Gynecol 1999;94(3):348–51.
40. Unger JB, Meeks GR. Vaginal hysterectomy in women with history of previous cesarean delivery. Am J Obstet Gynecol 1998;179(6 Pt 1):1473–8.
41. Kovac SR, Barhan S, Lister M, et al. Guidelines for the selection of the route of hysterectomy: application in a resident clinic population. Am J Obstet Gynecol 2002;187(6):1521–7.
42. Blandon RE, Bharucha AE, Melton LJ, et al. Incidence of pelvic floor repair after hysterectomy: A population-based cohort study. Am J Obstet Gynecol 2007; 197(6):664.e1–7.
43. Altman D, Falconer C, Cnattingius S, et al. Pelvic organ prolapse surgery following hysterectomy on benign indications. Am J Obstet Gynecol 2008; 198(5):572.e1–6.
44. Dällenbach P, Kaelin-Gambirasio I, Dubuisson JB, et al. Risk factors for pelvic organ prolapse repair after hysterectomy. Obstet Gynecol 2007;110(3):625–32.
45. Burkett D, Horwitz J, Kennedy V, et al. Assessing current trends in resident hysterectomy training. Female Pelvic Med Reconstr Surg 2011;17(5):210–4.

Cesarean Hysterectomy and Uterine-Preserving Alternatives

Christopher Kevin Huls, MD, MSc[a,b,c],*

KEYWORDS

- Cesarean • Hysterectomy • Postpartum • Hemorrhage • Atony • Previa • Accreta
- Conservative

KEY POINTS

- Postpartum hemorrhage remains a primary cause of maternal morbidity and mortality.
- Major causes of postpartum hemorrhage are atony, laceration, invasive placentation, sepsis, and coagulopathy.
- Management of postpartum hemorrhage requires an understanding of available medical and surgical treatments at each facility and a plan of care on how to access regional referral centers.
- Early identification of patients with clinically significant bleeding and prompt treatment to prevent the most likely complications is recommended.
- Multidisciplinary teams improve care by providing a systematic approach to postpartum complications, many of which have a common endpoint of hysterectomy or uterine-preserving techniques.

BACKGROUND

Peripartum hysterectomy is the removal of the uterine corpus at the time of delivery or during the immediate postpartum period. No commonly accepted definition places a limit on when the period ends. When performed at the time of cesarean delivery, it is termed a *cesarean hysterectomy*. A *postpartum hysterectomy* is performed after delivery of the fetus, with studies varying on whether a hysterectomy is performed within 24 hours, during the same hospitalization for delivery, or within the 6-week postpartum period.

Disclosure Statement: There are no relevant financial or research disclosures related to the writing of this article. The author has nothing to disclose.
[a] Department of Obstetrics and Gynecology, Banner University Medical Center, 1111 E McDowell, Phoenix, AZ, USA; [b] Department of Obstetrics and Gynecology, University of Arizona, Phoenix, AZ, USA; [c] Phoenix Perinatal Associates of Mednax, Inc., 1840 South Stapley Drive, Suite 131, Mesa, AZ 85204, USA
* Phoenix Perinatal Associates of Mednax, Inc., 1840 South Stapley Drive, Suite 131, Mesa, AZ 85204.
E-mail address: Kevin_Huls@pediatrix.com

Obstet Gynecol Clin N Am 43 (2016) 517–538
http://dx.doi.org/10.1016/j.ogc.2016.04.010
0889-8545/16/$ – see front matter © 2016 Elsevier Inc. All rights reserved.

The incidence of peripartum hysterectomy is on the rise.[1] Bateman and colleagues[1] performed a national cross-sectional study looking at more than 56 million deliveries from 1994 to 2007 and reported an increase in the overall rate from 71.6 to 82.6 per 100,000 deliveries. During that time, the rate of hysterectomy for abnormal placentation increased by 23%, from 32.9 to 40.5 per 100,000 deliveries, and uterine atony by 130%, from 11.2 to 25.9 per 100,000 deliveries. Hysterectomies not related to abnormal placentation, atony, delayed hemorrhage, or uterine rupture decreased during that period.[1] In the past, commonly accepted indications for hysterectomy included definitive treatment aimed to control bleeding or infection and even sterilization. Uterine atony and abnormal placentation continue to be common indications after vaginal delivery, primary cesarean, or repeat cesarean.[1–3] The contemporary use of hysterectomy indicators was detailed by the Maternal-Fetal Medicine Units Network looking at cesarean hysterectomy in a cohort of cesarean deliveries.[2] The most common indication for hysterectomy in their study was placenta accreta, which was the indication in 38.2% of the hysterectomies; other indications are listed in **Table 1**.[2] There were often measures taken to avoid hysterectomy, including uterine artery ligation (48%), ovarian artery ligation (20%), uterine packing (6%), hypogastric artery ligation (5%) oxytocin (9%), and uterine tamponade (14%).[2]

Adverse events related to peripartum hysterectomy are substantial.[3,4] The most common injury is to the bladder, which occurs in 9% of peripartum hysterectomies and only 1% of nonobstetric hysterectomies.[3,5] Other common risks include ureteral injury, hemorrhage, wound complications, and venous thromboembolism, which are increased with peripartum hysterectomies.[3] The risk of death with a peripartum hysterectomy is 1% (odds ratio [OR] 14.4; 95% CI, 9.84–20.98) compared with 0.04% for nonobstetric hysterectomy.[3] The risk of perioperative mortality, however, is 71% lower in high-volume centers compared with low-volume centers.[4]

Hysterectomy is a shared endpoint for postpartum hemorrhage after vaginal or cesarean delivery that is complicated by uterine atony, placental invasion, uterine rupture, leiomyomas, laceration extension, coagulopathy, or sepsis.[1,6] The techniques to manage these complications overlap and are often identified by recognizing unexpected bleeding or hemorrhage. Systematic protocols for postpartum hemorrhage

Table 1
Common indicators for peripartum hysterectomy

Indication	Wright et al,[3] 2010[a] Overall (%)	Shellhaas et al,[2] 2009[b] Overall (%)	Primary Cesarean Delivery (%)	Repeat Cesarean Delivery (%)
Placenta accreta	36.2	38.2	16.3	54.7
Atony	31.2	34.4	52.5	20.8
Cervical cancer	N/A	7.0	11.3	3.8
Uterine rupture	1.3	5.4	2.5	7.5
Leiomyoma	7.1	4.8	7.5	2.8
Extension	1.2	1.1	2.5	0.0
Other	N/A	9.1	7.5	10.4

[a] From vaginal deliveries and cesarean deliveries.
[b] From cesareans, primary cesarean, and repeat cesarean deliveries.
 Data from Wright JD, Devine P, Shah M, et al. Morbidity and mortality of peripartum hysterectomy. Obstet Gynecol 2010;115:1187–93; and Shellhaas CS, Gilbert S, Landon MB, et al. The frequency and complication rates of hysterectomy accompanying cesarean delivery. Obstet Gynecol 2009;114(2 Pt 1):224–9.

emphasize uterine atony as the most likely cause for bleeding and may not distinguish management based on diagnosis until unresponsive to initial therapy.[7,8] Conservative or uterine-preserving management refers to the management of peripartum complications by any method that avoids hysterectomy, which is intended to reduce the risk of complications and is generally the initial management for many of these indications.[6–9]

POSTPARTUM HEMORRHAGE

Hemorrhage remains a significant cause of maternal mortality worldwide and is currently the cause in 27% of all maternal deaths.[10] From 1987 to 2006, the percentage of deaths in the United States attributed to hemorrhage decreased and is currently responsible for 11.4% of maternal mortalities.[11] It is the 4th leading cause of mortality in the United States and the leading cause worldwide.[10] In the United States, maternal mortality from hemorrhage occurred most frequently with ruptured ectopic (3%), other causes (2.1%), uterine atony (1.8%), abnormally invasive placentation (1.4%), uterine rupture (1.1%), abruption (1.1%), placenta previa (0.3%), retained products (0.2%), and coagulopathy (0.2%).[11]

Postpartum hemorrhage is typically defined by the amount of blood loss after delivery, which is a vaginal delivery, with greater than or equal to 500 mL, and cesarean section, with greater than or equal to 1000 mL. Reported mean blood loss approximates these cutoffs for each route of delivery. The incidence of postpartum hemorrhage is reported to be 1% with active management and up to 3% without.[12,13] The most common cause of postpartum hemorrhage is uterine atony,[7] although the rate of abnormally invasive placentation as a cause for postpartum hemorrhage is increasing.[1,6]

UTERINE ATONY

The effective treatment of uterine atony includes prophylactic administration of medications, prompt recognition of atony as a cause of bleeding, and immediate treatment. It is important to have a thorough understanding of the mechanism of action for each medication and to understand the contraindications to their use. A summary of the medications is included in **Table 2**. Uterine atony may be encountered at the time of vaginal delivery or cesarean delivery or may present as a delayed complication in the postpartum period.

SURGICAL SITE BLEEDING AND ARTERIAL LIGATION

The original description by O'Leary and O'Leary[14] used a suture to compress the uterine artery along its expected anatomic location in the lateral aspect of the broad ligament. The original report included 90 patients with 6 failures; included among the failures were 3 patients with placenta accreta.[14] They also theorized that in placenta previa, blood supply arising from cervical or vaginal branches, may not be sufficiently occluded with ligation of the uterine artery, which was consistent with their observations. Since the initial report, uterine artery ligation at the time of cesarean or laparotomy has been a simple and effective initial step. To place an O'Leary suture the following steps are recommended:

- The uterine artery is palpated along the lateral aspect of the lower uterine segment.
- While compressing the uterine artery, the uterine artery and broad ligament are retracted by the surgeon laterally.

Table 2
Uterotonics

Medication	Dose and Route	Frequency	Comments
Oxytocin (Pitocin)	10–40 U diluted in normal saline or lactated Ringer solution	Continuous infusion	1–6 min half-life
	10 U intramuscular or intramyometrial	One time, unclear when to repeat	3–5 min onset, duration 3–5 h, 2–3 h duration
Methylergonovine (Methergine)	0.2 mg intramuscular or intramyometrial	Every 2–4 h	Contraindicated if hypertensive
15-Methyl prostaglandin F_{2a} (carboprost [Hemabate])	0.25 mg intramuscular or intramyometrial	Every 15–90 min up to 8 doses	Contraindicated if asthma Common gastrointestinal side effects
Dinoprostone (Prostin E_2)	20 mg rectal or vaginal suppository	Every 2 h	May cause bronchospasm
Prostaglandin E_2 (dinoprostone [Cervidil, Prepidil])	1000-µg rectal suppository	One time	Side effects include fever

- A suture is passed from the anterior uterus to the posterior uterus 2 cm to 3 cm medial to the uterine artery superior to the bladder and without requiring a bladder flap.
- The suture is then passed posterior to anterior through an avascular window of the broad ligament.

Today an O'Leary suture is a standard tool of obstetricians to reduce blood loss from unexpected surgical bleeding and manage postpartum hemorrhage to prevent peripartum hysterectomy. Unexpected bleeding may occur during cesarean delivery from laceration of the uterine artery during extension of the hysterotomy incision, lateral or low placental implantation site bleeding, coagulopathy, large leiomyomas, and uterine atony. Postpartum hemorrhage that is unresponsive to initial medications, uterine tamponade, or genital tract lacerations may be converted to laparotomy, and often the first intervention is placement of an O'Leary suture.[6,15] Prophylactic use of an O'Leary suture for patients with a leiomyoma can also reduce blood loss, improve postoperative hemoglobin, and reduce leiomyoma size.[16] Complications of an O'Leary suture can include hematoma, bleeding, ureteral injury, or inadequate control of bleeding.

Hypogastric artery ligation, also known as internal iliac ligation, is used to control bleeding with postpartum hemorrhage.[6,15] Ligation of this vessel reduces the pulse pressure into the pelvic organs by 85%. There is a trend away from using this technique due to the risk of complications and lack of familiarity with the anatomy. Ligation of the hypogastric artery also precludes endovascular embolization beyond the hypogastric vessels. There is likely a need for using this technique at facilities without access to interventional radiologist.[2,6] If the operator is inexperienced with the technique, an experienced surgeon is recommended to assist. Performing this procedure involves the following:

- Open the anterior leaf of the broad ligament to identify the external iliac.
- Trace vessel to origin of common iliac. Identify the anterior division of the internal iliac.

- Use nonabsorbable suture to tie lateral to medial.
- Complications may involve ligation of the external iliac, which leads to loss of lower extremity pulses or injury to the internal iliac vein.

COMPRESSION SUTURES

The B-Lynch suture and other variations are designed to provide compression to the uterus by mechanical force. This technique may be used at the time of cesarean or during an exploratory laparotomy. The original description used a chromic suture, although a monofilament, such as a no. 1 poliglecaprone 25 suture, is less likely to cause trauma. A B-Lynch procedure is performed with the following steps:

- Placing a vertical anchoring suture in the lower uterine segment and at the corner of hysterotomy
- Pulling the suture superiorly and looping over the uterine fundus
- Placing a horizontal suture along the posterior aspect of the lower uterine segment
- Pulling the suture superiorly and looping over the uterine fundus
- Placing a second vertical anchoring suture across from the initial suture at the corner of the hysterotomy
- With compression from an assistant, tightening and tying the suture

There are other techniques that are similar in principle to the B-Lynch suture. Recent reviews concluded that the strength of evidence to evaluate effectiveness and harms of compression sutures is low.[9,15] As a secondary measure to control bleeding, success of the suture depends on the decrease in bleeding related to compression. If compression of the uterus by the surgeon or assistant does not seem effective in decreasing blood loss, then placement of a suture for that purpose is not likely to be successful, and consideration for other causes for bleeding, such as laceration, invasive placentation, and coagulopathy, is recommended.

UTERINE TAMPONADE

Uterine balloon catheters are designed to tamponade placental bleeding sites within the uterine cavity. This is most effective when the catheter is able to apply direct pressure to the bleeding site. Uterine balloon devices designed specifically for the tamponade of uterine bleeding after vaginal or cesarean delivery include the Foley catheter, Bakri balloon, B-T Cath device (Utah Medical Products Inc., Utah, USA), and the double-balloon Ebb device (Clinical Innovations, Utah, USA), which is also designed to tamponade cervical bleeding.[6,17] The Foley catheter may be instilled with 60 mL to 80 mL of saline, with placement of multiple catheters,[6] and the various balloon catheters have manufacturer limits on the amount of fluid recommended for each device. The Bakri balloon is recommended to be filled to 300 mL to 500 mL, although the devices can be filled with 300 mL to 1200 mL of fluid to distend the uterus.[6,17,18] To effectively exert pressure against a bleeding surface area, the balloon may require additional distension.[19] Ineffective use of the device can occur with distortion of the uterine cavity from anomalies or leiomyomas, retained placenta, expansion of the cavity by clot or debris, loss of uterine tone, or laceration extending into an open or intra-abdominal space may not allow the device to apply sufficient pressure to tamponade bleeding.

INTERVENTIONAL RADIOLOGY

Interventional radiology has remarkably advanced minimally invasive management of postpartum hemorrhage, placenta accreta, and pelvic abscess drainage. Endovascular embolization for postpartum hemorrhage allows rapid and selective control of bleeding.[6] A recent systematic review, which defined success as requiring no additional procedures, estimated an 89% to 91% success rate.[9,15] For patients with placental invasion or placenta accreta, success is reported with uterine artery, hypogastric artery, or aortic balloons as prophylactic treatment when placed prior to delivery and then insufflated after delivery if needed.[20–23] A drawback with preoperative placement is the need to expose the fetus to ionizing radiation and the need to transfer patients between the radiology suite and operating room,[24] although newly designed hybrid operating rooms eliminate the need to transfer unstable patients intraoperatively. It is also possible to place balloon catheters prior to delivery and then after delivery selective embolization is used. Uterine artery embolization is technically feasible in 97% of placenta accreta cases,[25] with reported decreases in blood loss and transfusion requirements.[25,26] This method is reportedly used by multidisciplinary teams, and improvement in select cases is also reported.[24,27] Complications with balloon catheters are reported and rupture of the vessels cited as the primary complication encountered.[21–24] A staged procedure that involves embolization after delivery holds promise for reducing blood loss and hysterectomy rate, but additional studies are needed.[28] One advantage of embolization is the ability to selectively embolize uterine arteries, hypogastric arteries, significant collateral arteries, or parasitized blood supply.

MASSIVE TRANSFUSION

Massive transfusion protocols were developed after recent military use.[29] It was recognized that significant morbidity and mortality occurred when bleeding continued after adequate replacement of red blood cells. After the initial blood loss, red blood cell replacement, and volume resuscitation, ongoing blood losses would continue and eventually other signs of coagulopathy would manifest. By early and systematic replacement of fresh frozen plasma and platelets, there is a decrease in significant and ongoing blood loss. Red blood cells acquired for storage are separated into packed red blood cells, plasma, cryoprecipitate, and platelets, and, therefore, the packed red blood cells are lacking sufficient coagulation proteins and platelets when used. The largest amount of stored proteins is in fresh frozen plasma.

The clotting cascade is extensive and involves multiple factors and platelets for coagulation.

- Initially tissue factor and factor VIIa bind to form a complex that activates factors X and IX.
- Factor Xa binds to complex with factor Va, which then activates prothrombin (factor II) to thrombin (factor IIa).
- Thrombin (factor IIa) activates fibrinogen to fibrin and promotes additional activation of factor V to factor Va. There is further amplification from thrombin (factor IIa) activating factor VIII, allowing factors IXa and VIIIa to complex. Thrombin (factor IIa) also activates factor XI to factor XIa, which amplifies activation of factor IX to IXa. Lastly, thrombin activates factor XIII to factor XIIIa, which cross-links fibrin polymers.

The guiding principle for massive transfusion protocols is to replace equal amounts of red blood cells, coagulation factors, and platelets. After the initial resuscitation of crystalloid and blood, transfusion of fresh frozen plasma and platelets are typically done in a 1:1:1 fashion, although the exact units may vary by institution.[29] Massive transfusion protocols have been implemented in obstetrics and used by many tertiary referral centers. It is important to identify how each facility manages massive transfusion protocols because variation exists, and there are many resource-lacking areas that do not have the capability to provide massive transfusions. Facilities that do not have the ability to provide massive transfusion need to identify at-risk patients and facilitate early and appropriate transfers of care prior to delivery.

ANTIFIBRINOLYTICS

Tranexamic acid is an antifibrinolytic medication used for preventing massive bleeding in the setting of hemorrhage, trauma, or menstrual bleeding and prior to procedures for patients with hemophilia. It is a synthetic analog of lysine, an amino acid that binds to lysine receptors on plasminogen or plasmin. The resultant effect prevents degradation of fibrin polymers. When used as a prophylactic medication, there is decreased blood loss at delivery (261.5 mL $\pm$ 146.8 mL vs 349.98 mL $\pm$ 188.85 mL; $P<.001$) and reduced postpartum hemorrhage at the time of vaginal delivery (relative risk [RR] 3.76; 95% CI, 1.27–11.15; $P = .01$).[30] A study of 144 patients evaluated use of tranexamic acid after a postpartum hemorrhage greater than 800 mL and found that there was less blood loss, shorter duration of bleeding, and less red blood cell transfusion.[31] A recent Cochrane review looked at 12 trials comprising 3285 patients and concluded that blood loss after either vaginal delivery or cesarean was decreased with tranexamic acid use even when routine uterotonics were used.[32] Further studies are needed to determine the optimal dosing regimen.

TOPICAL HEMOSTATIC AGENTS

Topical hemostatic agents take advantage of their biochemical and chemical properties to control persistent bleeding arising from large surfaces or coagulopathy. In pregnancy the increased edema makes tissue more friable and likely to bleed with extensive manipulation. Coagulopathy can result from postpartum hemorrhage; severe preeclampsia; hemolysis, elevated liver enzymes, and low platelets (HELLP) syndrome; thrombocytopenia; abruption; sepsis; and uterine rupture. At that point, the patient lacks essential components to form clot, and after an initial activation of the clotting cascade, the fibrinolytic system becomes more active, which quickly breaks down the formation of any clot. Adequate treatment with uterotonics, compression, or arterial ligation does not effectively address the underlying cause of ongoing blood loss once coagulopathy is present. Topical agents with fibrinogen and thrombin allow clot to form at the application site even when coagulopathy persists. Agents are available in a variety of application methods, which includes powders, sheets, liquids, and sprays, which can be applied over a wide area.

There are several extensive reviews available that discuss the use of hemostatic agents to control intraoperative bleeding.[33] The agents most commonly used in obstetric are summarized in **Table 3**. The initial use and experience of these agents were from trauma, cardiovascular surgery, orthopedic surgery, urology, and neurosurgery. The effectiveness of these agents in preventing the need for hysterectomy is unknown, but case reports on products like combat gauze seem promising.[34] Despite currently lacking data to guide use, these agents are valuable approaches to control obstetric blood loss and may hold promise for uterine preservation.

Not all topical hemostatic agents may be safe to use during pregnancy. Bone wax is used for controlling bleeding along the surface of the bone by occlusion of bleeding channels within bone. Although this may not be encountered during obstetric surgery, its use after orthopedic trauma is worth discussing. A study in rats identified teratogenic potential when bone wax was used on pregnant rates.[35]

Table 3
Topical hemostatic agents for use during pregnancy

Product	Mechanism	Types of Bleeding	Disadvantages	Trade Names
Absorbable agents				
Gelatin foam	Physical matrix • Film • Sponge • Powder	Small vessel bleeding Hemostatic plug wrapped in oxidized cellulose Absorbed by the body within 6 wk Nonantigenic Neutral pH, can use with biologics	Swells with hydration and can cause damage in small spaces Embolization if in intravascular space	Gelfilm Gelfoam
Oxidized cellulose	Physical matrix Low pH	Antimicrobial effect from low pH Easy to handle, does not stick to instruments Dissolves within 6 wk	Low pH • Inactivates other biologics, such as thrombin • Inflammation	Surgicel Fibrillar Surgicel Nu-Knit
Microfibrillar collagen	Adheres and activates platelets	Control wide areas of bleeding Effective in heparinized conditions	Decreased efficacy with thrombocytopenia Caution with recollection devices because product passes through filter Adheres to instruments/surgical gloves	Avitene Avitene Flour Endo Avitene Avitene Ultrafoam Avitene UltraWrap Instat Helitene Helistat

Biologic agents

Agent	Description	Characteristics	Brand names
Thrombin	Converts fibrinogen to fibrin Activates clotting factors	Minor bleeding from capillaries, small venules unresponsive to pressure Rapid acting	High immunogenicity with bovine derivatives	Thrombin-JMI (bovine), Evithrom (human derived) Recothrom Recothrom (recombinant human)
Thrombin with gelatin	Gelatin cross-links into matrix to tamponade Thrombin effect	Moderate arterial bleeding due to gelatin tamponade effect	Required contact with blood Increases size rapidly after application	Floseal
Fibrin sealant	Thrombin and fibrinogen mix at application site Thrombin cleaves fibrinogen to fibrin	Effective with heparinization Venous oozing from denuded surfaces	Time to prepare	Tisseel Evicel Crosseal
Platelet gel	Microfibrillar collagen and thrombin combined with patients plasma, which contains fibrinogen and platelets	Arterial and venous use. Utilizes patient's platelets, facilitate tissue regeneration	Caution with blood scavenging systems	Vitagel

ACTIVATED FACTORS

Activated factors are available, and approved by the Food and Drug Administration for use in promoting hemostasis for patients with acquired or inherited defects in coagulation. Recombinant factor VII is approved for use in patients with hemophilia, autoantibodies to factors VIII or IX, and congenital deficiency of factor VII. Of all of the available activated factors, factor VIIa has been used off-label to control bleeding from postpartum hemorrhage or surgical bleeding. Lavigne-Lissalde and colleagues[36] studied a total of 84 women and treated 42 patients with a single dose of recombinant factor VIIa or standard care for patients with postpartum hemorrhage unresponsive to uterotonics. There were 22 of 42 (52%) patients who required additional therapies when treated with factor VIIa compared with 39 of 42 (93%) patients with standard care who required additional therapies.[36] There were no deaths, but there were 2 venous thrombotic events after treatment.

INVASIVE PLACENTATION, MORBIDLY ADHERENT PLACENTATION, PLACENTA ACCRETA, PLACENTA INCRETA, AND PLACENTA PERCRETA

Placenta accreta is a risk factor for maternal morbidity and mortality. The Centers for Disease Control and Prevention in the United States reported that from 2006 to 2010 the risk of maternal death from placenta accreta was 1.4% of all obstetric deaths.[11] The incidence of placenta accreta seems to be increasing for referral centers, with a reported rate of 1 in 4027 prior to 1980 that increased to 1 in 533 in a single referral center.[37] Another large multicenter study of 25 academic centers found the rate of morbidly adherent placentation to be 1 in 731.[38] In contrast to referral centers, a large health care delivery system reported only 1 death from placenta accreta in a review of 1,461,270 deliveries.[39]

Morbidly adherent placentation refers to the clinical recognition of delayed placental separation during the third stage of labor that is often associated with placenta accreta, placenta increta, or placenta percreta. Placenta accreta is invasion of the trophoblasts into the myometrium with failure to transform maternal spiral arteries and form Nitabuch layer, which is responsible for separating during the third stage of labor. Placenta increta is trophoblastic invasion deep into the myometrium. Placenta percreta is invasion of trophoblast up to and beyond the uterine serosa.

Risk factors for placenta accreta are present in a majority of patients who are diagnosed with the disorder, although this is not required. The strongest risk factor is placenta previa with a risk of 3%,[37] and the risk for placenta accreta increases with the number of prior cesareans.[40,41] When previa is present, there is an 11% risk of placenta accreta with 1 prior cesarean, 40% with 2 prior cesareans and 60% with 3 or more prior cesareans.[40,41] Even when there is no placenta previa, the risk for placenta accreta increases with the number of prior cesareans, reaching 4.7% with 6 or more prior cesareans.[40] The risk for placenta accreta is associated with several conditions, many of which involve injury to the endometrium or myometrium and include myomectomy, uterine curettage, endometrial ablation,[42] Asherman syndrome, leiomyoma, and pelvic radiation.[43] Other risk factors include age greater than 35 years,[37] multiparity,[37] abortion,[37] and cesarean scar ectopic.[44,45]

Understanding the definitions and histopathology of placenta accreta, placenta increta, and placenta percreta helps explain the antenatal diagnostic criteria used to diagnose abnormal placentation. Trophoblasts seem more heterogeneous in the transformation of spiral arteries, particularly when implantation occurs in areas of endometrial or myometrial damage. A study evaluated vessel diameter size from patients with abnormal placentation and compared this with controls. They identified greater heterogeneity of vessel distribution containing fewer capillaries with larger capillary diameters, and larger diameter vessels compared with controls.[46] Normal placentation seems to have a more uniform distribution of small, medium, and large vessel diameters, and the overall total area occupied by vessels was not different between placenta increta and controls.[46] These changes can help explain the ultrasound findings associated with abnormal placentation. In a multivariate analysis, ultrasounds with placental lacunae (OR 1.5; 95% CI, 1.4–1.6), loss of the retroplacental hypoechoic zone (OR, 2.4; 95% CI, 1.1–4.9), or abnormal color Doppler (OR, 2.1; 95% CI, 1.8–2.4) may be more likely in patients with the disorder.[47] The use of ultrasound findings to increase the sensitivity or specificity of detecting abnormally invasive placentation is highly dependent on the clinical history,[48] and MRI has similar diagnostic capability.[49]

Reported findings associated with abnormally invasive placentation are

- Cesarean scar ectopic
- Loss of retroplacental hypoechoic zone
- Vascular lacunae or large venous lakes, which may have turbulent flow
- Irregular serosal border and bladder interface
- Myometrial thickness along retroplacental area less than 1 mm
- Large coalescing vascular flow within the placenta

Antenatal diagnosis of placenta accreta, placenta increta, and placenta percreta occurs in only 50% to 53% of patients prior to delivery.[38,50] Surprisingly, 18% of patients diagnosed with invasive placentation are nulliparous, and 37% have no prior cesarean deliveries.[38] When the diagnosis is suspected antenatally, there is likely to be less blood loss (2750 vs 6100 mL; $P = .008$) and less need for transfusion (59 vs 94%; $P = .014$) and fewer attempts to remove placenta.[50] **Table 4** provides the distribution of outcomes for patients diagnosed prior to delivery and those at the time of delivery. One possible explanation for the difference in outcomes is that when placental invasion is more clinically significant, there may be more than 1 associated finding for invasive placentation, which may also indicate deeper invasion, and result in significant complications being experienced at delivery.

Knowing that placenta accreta is suspected allows referral to centers of excellence for placenta accreta.[51] The advantages of such centers are the expertise, experience, and dedication of resources that are needed in managing complex cases of placenta accreta. Centers often have a defined multidisciplinary team, which is associated with

Table 4
Outcomes observed when placenta accreta, placenta increta, or placenta percreta is suspected antenatally

	Antenatal Diagnosis Prior to Delivery	Undiagnosed Prior to Delivery
Large blood loss (>2750 mL)	33%	19%
Hysterectomy	92%	45%
Admission to ICU	39%	22%
Gestational age at delivery (wk)	35.6% (33.6–36.9)	37.8 (35.4–39.6)
Neonatal ventilator support within 24 h	28.6% (18.9–38.2)	10.8 (3.7–17.9)
Neonatal ICU admission	65.5% (55.3–75.6)	33.8 (23.0–44.6)

Data are percentages with CI (5%–95%).
Data from Bailit JL, Grobman WA, Rice MM, et al. Morbidly Adherent placenta treatments and outcomes. Obstet Gynecol 2015;125:683–9.

reduced blood loss and morbidity.[52–54] There is often a systematic approach to treating patients, which can include administration of antenatal corticosteroids, timing for delivery, use of ureteral stents, skin incision, uterine incision, involvement of interventional radiology, decisions and counseling for expectant management or uterine preservation, consultation with surgical specialists, management of massive transfusion, and ICU support.[4,52–55] Suggestions for criteria to designate a center of excellence for placenta accreta are in **Box 1**.[51]

A center of excellence serves to function as regionalized care to prevent complications and improve outcomes. Appropriate management focuses on making an accurate prenatal diagnosis, access to consultants, and predelivery planning.[27,54] Centers are experienced in making clinical care plans for complex invasive placentation,[24,54] planning preterm delivery,[56] and when to perform embolization.[26,54]

Criteria when considering referral to a center of excellence for placenta accreta have been proposed and are found in **Box 2**.[51] A patient is suspected of having a placenta accreta either from clinical risk factors or from sonographic factors on prenatal ultrasound. Clinical risk factors include current or prior placenta previa, current or prior cesarean delivery, multiple previous cesarean deliveries, history endometrial ablation, previous uterine surgeries, and first-trimester or second-trimester bleeding, with other risk factors for placenta accreta.[37,40,41,44,51,57] Ultrasound sonographic risk factors include identification of an abnormal placenta, abnormal uterine shape, abnormal vascularity of the myometrial wall, or current or previous cesarean scar ectopic.[44,45,47,48,51]

UNEXPECTED PLACENTA ACCRETA

Placenta accreta may not be suspected prior to delivery in approximately 47% to 50% of cases.[38,50] Clinical recognition after vaginal delivery is a delayed separation

---

Box 1
Suggested criteria for center of excellence for placenta accreta

1. Multidisciplinary team
   a. Experienced maternal-fetal medicine physician or obstetrician
   b. Imaging experts (ultrasound and MRI)
   c. Pelvic surgeon (ie, gynecologic oncology or urogynecology)
   d. Anesthesiologist (ie, obstetric or cardiac anesthesia)
   e. Urologist
   f. Trauma or general surgeon
   g. Interventional radiologist
   h. Neonatologist

2. ICU and facilities
   a. Interventional radiology
   b. Surgical or medical ICU
      i. 24-Hour availability of intensive care specialists
   c. Neonatal ICU
      i. Gestational age appropriate for neonate

3. Blood services
   a. Massive transfusion capabilities
   b. Cell saver and perfusionists
   c. Experience and access to alternative blood products
   d. Guidance of transfusion medicine specialists or blood bank pathologists

From Silver RM, Fox KA, Barton JR, et al. Center of excellence for placenta accreta. Am J Obstet Gynecol 2015;213(6):755–60; with permission.

Box 2
Criteria for consideration of delivery in center of excellence for placenta accreta

1. Suspicion for placenta accreta on sonogram

2. Placenta previa with abnormal ultrasound appearance

3. Placenta previa with 3 or more prior cesarean deliveries

4. History of classic cesarean delivery and anterior placentation

5. History or endometrial ablation or pelvic irradiation

6. Inability to adequately evaluate or exclude findings suspicious for placenta accreta in women with risk factors for placenta accreta

7. Any other reason for suspicion of placenta accreta

From Silver RM, Fox KA, Barton JR, et al. Center of excellence for placenta accreta. Am J Obstet Gynecol 2015;213(6):755–60; with permission.

---

unresponsive to uterotonics and gentle traction. Expulsion of the placenta may also occur with ensuing postpartum hemorrhage unresponsive to uterotonics and no evidence of genital tract laceration, coagulopathy, leiomyoma, or uterine inversion. During exploratory laparotomy or cesarean delivery, findings on the serosal surface, such as large varicosities, distended lower uterine segment with bulging, or direct extension of placenta onto the uterine surface, bladder, or pelvic sidewalls may provide clues although may be nondescript with placenta accreta.[51] **Fig. 1** is an example of an anterior wall placenta percreta, and **Fig. 2** is a lateral wall placenta percreta. A proposed management strategy is suggested and is seen in **Box 3**.

The delivering physician must decide whether to proceed with delivery or transfer based on maternal medical needs need like excessive bleeding or clinical instability, rather than based on fetal indication. If a delivery site is not equipped or prepared, then if at all possible the patient should be transferred to a referral center.[4] Care for the mother over the fetus still remains paramount. If delivery needs to proceed, then avoid disturbing or removing the placenta by using a fundal or posterior uterine

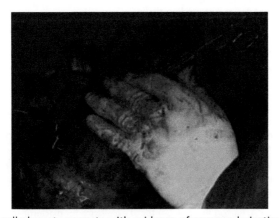

Fig. 1. Anterior wall placenta percreta with evidence of neovascularization across the uterine serosa, distortion of the serosa, and varicosities on the surface.

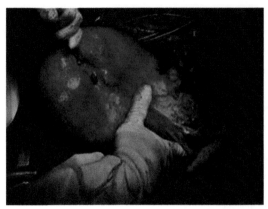

Fig. 2. Lateral wall placenta percreta with serosal vessels and distortion of the lower uterine segment.

incision if needed.[50] If available, uterine mapping with an ultrasound and sterile probe cover may assist in placing a uterine incision opposite to placental location. The maternal abdominal incision may require a vertical midline incision or creation of a T-shaped incision. Avoid manipulating the uterus after delivery of the neonate and ligate the umbilical cord close to placental insertion with an absorbable suture, which may be left in utero for conservative management.[50] Close the hysterotomy site with an absorbable suture and ensure hemostasis at incision site. Oxytocin may be used to ensure uterine tone, although it is unclear if this increases partial separation of the placenta. If the patient is then stable, transfer may be facilitated at this time.

Box 3
Management of unsuspected placenta percreta discovered at laparotomy

- Delay uterine incision if survey seems abnormal
  - Distorted or ballooned lower uterine segment
  - Blood vessels on uterine serosa
  - Invasion into bladder or surrounding tissue

- Assess location and extent of placental invasion visually and by ultrasound

- Evaluate for presence of active bleeding

- Inquire about available resources: blood or blood products, surgical consultants, necessary equipment, and location

- If patient is stable and facility is not currently prepared
  - Cover uterus with warm laparotomy packs and await assistance and supplies before proceeding with intervention.
  - Close fascial incision, place staples in skin, and consider transfer to tertiary facility with experience in management of placenta percreta.

- If patient is actively bleeding, apply local pressure to bleeding areas (other than areas where placental tissue is at risk), then prepare for hysterotomy and delivery followed by surgical or conservative management of placenta percreta.

From Silver RM, Fox KA, Barton JR, et al. Center of excellence for placenta accreta. Am J Obstet Gynecol 2015;213(6):755–60; with permission.

CONSERVATIVE MANAGEMENT

Conservative management of placenta accreta is used to describe management without using a hysterectomy at delivery and involves expectantly managing patients, which may require adjunctive surgical or medical treatment. The largest and most complete study on using conservative management as the primary strategy was reported by Sentilles and colleagues.[58] They looked 167 of 311 patients diagnosed with placenta accreta from 25 institutions in France where hysterectomy or cesarean hysterectomy was not planned and reported their observations. They were able to successfully treat 78.4% of their patients with expectant management, but significant morbidity was encountered.[58] Hysterectomy occurred in 21.6% (36 patients), with half resulting from primary postpartum hemorrhage at delivery, and delayed hysterectomy occurred at a median of 22 days.[58] Morbidity for the cohort included[59] the need for extensive antibiotics (32.3%), transfusion (41.9%), ICU (25.7%), and secondary postpartum hemorrhage (10.8%), with 1 maternal death.[58] Complications requiring hysterectomy include secondary postpartum hemorrhage, sepsis, vesicouterine fistula, uterine necrosis, arteriovenous malformation, or if indicated by maternal request.[58,60] Other reported complications include disseminated intravascular coagulation.[58,59,61]

When a placenta remains in situ and bleeding remains minimal, no further procedures are required and expectant management may be pursued. Uterotonics may be used initially to maintain uterine tone, which can assist with bleeding at the hysterotomy site and is commonly used for retained placenta as an initial measure. For expectant management, the abdominal incision is closed and close surveillance is done in the postpartum period. No standardized approach to postpartum follow-up exists but typically involves frequent visits, ultrasound, and laboratory work to identify resolution and complications.

Methotrexate use has become standard first-line treatment of early ectopic pregnancies and is selectively used for medical management of cesarean scar ectopic pregnancies.[45] Methotrexate acts on rapidly dividing cells, but in the third trimester the placenta is no longer rapidly dividing. This likely explains why methotrexate has not been demonstrated to show added benefit for conservative management of placenta accreta. Routine use of methotrexate for placenta accreta is not recommended at this time.[62]

Removal of the placenta may occur because invasive placentation was not suspected, only a focal area was suspected, premature separation of the placenta, or when multidisciplinary teams at centers of excellence are attempting to utilize methods for uterine preservation. Perioperative placement of uterine artery balloon catheters may improve outcomes.[20,21] Placement of artery balloon catheter is technically possible in the iliac arteries[22] and aorta,[23] but improvements in maternal outcomes are uncertain. Prophylactic uterine artery embolization is possible after delivery and helpful for reducing blood loss and for uterine preservation but may be limited based on availability.[25,28] Bakri balloon placement is reported if the placenta is removed, which is passed from intra-abdominal route to vagina with an assistant pulling the infusion ports through to the vagina. The balloon is filled with water, traction applied, and the hysterotomy may be closed over the balloon.

CESAREAN HYSTERECTOMY PROCEDURE

Performing a peripartum hysterectomy involves a similar approach to hysterectomy in nonobstetric patients. Preparations include positioning of the patient in a manner that allows the operator to accomplish the goals of the surgery. This may include either a supine position or dorsal lithotomy position.

Antibiotic prophylaxis reduces the risk of surgical site infection when given preoperatively. In a Cochrane review of 95 studies, use of antibiotics reduced the risk of wound infection (RR 0.4; 95% CI, 0.35–0.46), endometritis (RR 0.38; 95% CI, 0.34–0.42), and serious maternal infection (RR 0.31; 95% CI, 0.2–0.49).[63] The most commonly used regimen was cephazolin, 2 g intravenous. An alternative regimen was used for patients with a penicillin allergy, most commonly clindamycin, 900 mg, plus gentamicin, 5 mg/kg. A recent study on surgical site skin preparation demonstrated superiority of chlorhexidine-alcohol with a 4% risk of associated surgical-site infection compared with iodine-alcohol with a risk of 7.3% (RR 0.55; 95% CI, 0.34–0.90).[64]

The choice of incision is based on the need for anticipated complications during surgery. A Pfannenstiel incision is commonly performed for routine primary or repeat cesarean delivery or may be used for nonobstetric abdominal hysterectomy. The disadvantage with this type of incision is limited access and visualization to the upper pelvis and abdomen. A vertical skin incision is chosen to minimize bleeding, reduce entry time, provide adequate exposure to the upper abdomen, and allow extension of the incision if required. A vertical skin incision may be preferred in the settings of coagulopathy, need for emergent delivery, and placenta previa, which may preclude delivery of the fetus through a transverse uterine incision. For a situation in which a hysterectomy is planned, or the surgery is expected to be difficult, a vertical skin incision may be more advantageous.

TECHNIQUE

A decision to proceed with hysterectomy may be based on a patient's desire for future fertility, partial placental separation, active bleeding, presence of placenta percreta extending to pelvic structures, availability of resources, role as a referral center or center of excellence, access to adequate blood products, and clinical instability. The steps of a peripartum hysterectomy are the same as for nonobstetric hysterectomy:

- Separation of round ligament
- Separation of broad ligament (**Figs. 3** and **4**)
- Dissection of bladder and perivesicular space
- Palpation, clamping, and separation of the cardinal ligament and uterine arteries (**Figs. 5** and **6**)

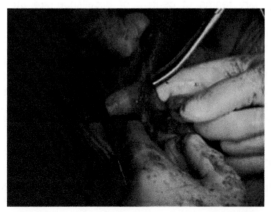

Fig. 3. Separation of broad ligament. An avascular window is identified and with electrocautery the window is created. Surgical clamps or free ties may be used to suture ligate.

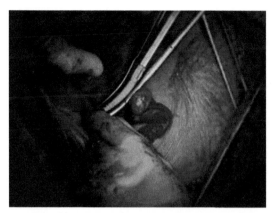

Fig. 4. Clamping across broad ligament. Clamps are placed across the pedicle of the broad ligament created by the avascular window. This may be further ligated with suture for additional hemostasis.

- Separation of the uterosacral ligament (**Fig. 7**)
- Closure of the vaginal cuff

Pregnancy changes may further complicate surgery, especially from the increased uterine blood flow during pregnancy. There is an approximate 10-fold to 30-fold increase in uterine blood flow that approximates 450 mL/min to 650 mL/min by term.[65,66] The risk for sudden and catastrophic blood loss is much greater during late gestation than for traditional hysterectomy. Tissue fragility and edema is increased, which makes handling tissue more difficult. Normal anatomic relationships to other structures may be displaced. The ureters may be tortuous, distended, and with significant hydroureter or hydronephrosis. The enlarged uterus itself poses challenges to visualization and palpation.

Traditionally surgical techniques relied on double clamping and double tying of suture for a peripartum hysterectomy. Newly advanced techniques with vessel sealing

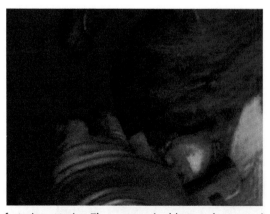

Fig. 5. Palpation of uterine arteries. The surgeon is able to palpate uterine arteries prior to placing clamps across the uterine arteries. This is also done to ensure integrity of the myometrium before placing clamps. Placing the clamp may traumatize the tissue or disrupt the placenta if there is little myometrium present.

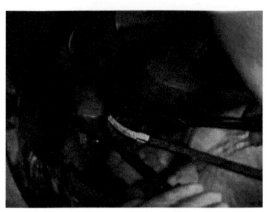

Fig. 6. Clamping across uterine arteries. Clamps are placed across the uterine arteries. Two clamps are placed for compression and control of additional bleeding.

devices (LigaSure [Medtronic, Minneapolis, MN]) allows for coagulation, desiccation, and sealing of vascular pedicles. The use of vessel sealing devices limits tissue trauma and replaces 1 step for clamping and tying the tissue. These devices are considered most effective with vessels less than or equal to 7 mm. One study compared surgical outcomes for peripartum hysterectomy when the LigaSure device was used and when it was not. It reported less operative time, less blood loss, and reduced incidence of massive blood loss during the procedure with the use of LigaSure.[67]

Completion of the hysterectomy with either a subtotal or total hysterectomy is operator dependent. The goal of surgery is to achieve hemostasis, reduce infection, remove necrotic material or abscess, remove the placenta when morbidly adhered, and reduce maternal morbidity. The goal is not to remove the cervix unless it is the cause of bleeding, requires histologic evaluation, or can be safely removed without compromising hemostasis. A survey for possible injuries, evaluation of other areas of bleeding, use of topical hemostatic agents, assessing the integrity of the bladder,

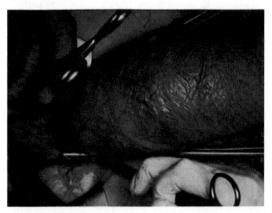

Fig. 7. Clamping across the uterosacrals. Once bladder dissection is achieved, clamping across the uterosacral ligaments below placenta percreta and placenta previa allows removal of specimen as either subtotal or total hysterectomy.

and possible removal of the fallopian tubes to reduce ovarian cancer is also recommended.

SUMMARY

Hysterectomy is an uncommon procedure for the obstetric patient. It is a procedure reserved to be lifesaving and the indications for its use are associated with maternal morbidity and mortality.

- Hysterectomy is a final endpoint for postpartum hemorrhage protocols, but the success of protocols requires early identification and active management of bleeding patients.
- Postpartum hemorrhage from uterine atony remains the most common indication for peripartum hysterectomy, although there is now an increased incidence of abnormally invasive placenta accreta, placenta increta, and placenta percreta.
- Abnormally invasive placentation is diagnosed antenatally in 50% to 53% of patients requiring hysterectomy. Antenatal diagnosis of this disorder improves outcomes.
- Uterotonics, balloon tamponade, and postpartum hemorrhage protocols remain the first steps in managing postpartum hemorrhage.
- Postpartum hemorrhage unresponsive to uterotonics and compression may be caused by genital tract laceration, coagulopathy, or abnormally invasive placentation.
- Early and aggressive use of massive transfusion protocols may prevent large blood volume loss.
- Multidisciplinary teams along with improvements in interventional radiology achieve improved outcomes for complicated postpartum patients.

REFERENCES

1. Bateman BT, Mhyre JM, Callaghan WM, et al. Peripartum hysterectommy in the United States: nationwide 14 year experience. Am J Obstet Gynecol 2012;206: 63.e1–8.
2. Shellhaas CS, Gilbert S, Landon MB, et al. The frequency and complication rates of hysterectomy accompanying cesarean delivery. Obstet Gynecol 2009;114(2 Pt 1):224–9.
3. Wright JD, Devine P, Shah M, et al. Morbidity and mortality of peripartum hysterectomy. Obstet Gynecol 2010;115:1187–93.
4. Wright JD, Herzog TJ, Shah M, et al. Regionalization of care for obstetric hemorrhage and its effect on maternal mortality. Obstet Gynecol 2010;115:1194–200.
5. Clark EA, Silver RM. Long-term maternal morbidity associated with repeat cesarean delivery. Am J Obstet Gynecol 2011;205(6 Suppl):S2–10.
6. American College of Obstetricians and Gynecologists. Postpartum hemorrhage. Practice bulletin 76. Obstet Gynecol 2006;108:1039–47.
7. Shields LE, Wiesner S, Fulton J, et al. Comprehensive maternal hemorrhage protocols reduce the use of blood products and improve patient safety. Am J Obstet Gynecol 2015;212(3):272–80.
8. Einerson BD, Miller ES, Grobman WA. Does a postpartum hemorrhage patient safety program result in sustained changes in management and outcomes? Am J Obstet Gynecol 2015;212(2):140–4.
9. Mousa HA, Blum J, Abou El Senoun G, et al. Treatment for primary postpartum haemorrhage. Cochrane Database Syst Rev 2014;(2):CD003249.

10. Say L, Chou A, Tuncalp O, et al. Global causes of maternal death: a WHO systematic analysis. Lancet 2014;2(6):e323–33.

11. Creanga AA, Berg CJ, Syverson C, et al. Pregnancy-related mortality in the United States 2006-2010. Obstet Gynecol 2015;125(1):5–12.

12. Rogers J, Wood J, McCandlish R, et al. Active versus expectant management of third stage of labour: the Hinchingbrooke randomised controlled trial. Lancet 1999;351(9104):693–9.

13. Prendiville WJ, Elbourne D, McDonald SJ. Active versus expectant management in the third stage of labour. Cochrane Database Syst Rev 2000;(3):CD000007.

14. O'Leary JL, O'Leary JA. Uterine artery ligation for control of postcesarean section hemorrhage. Obstet Gynecol 1974;43(6):849–53.

15. Sathe NA, Likis FE, Young JL, et al. Procedures and uterine-sparing surgeries for managing postpartum hemorrhage: a systematic review. Obstet Gynecol Surv 2016;71(2):99–113.

16. Liu WM, Wang PH, Tang WL, et al. Uterine artery ligation for treatment of pregnant women with uterine leiomyomas who are undergoing cesarean section. Fertil Steril 2006;86(2):423–8.

17. Dildy GA, Belfort MA, Adair D, et al. Initial experience with a dual-balloon catheter for the management of postpartum hemorrhage. Am J Obstet Gynecol 2014;210: 136.e1–6.

18. Bakri YN, Amri A, Abdul Jabbar F. Tamponade-balloon for obstetrical bleeding. Int J Gynaecol Obstet 2001;74(2):139–42.

19. Kaya B, Tuten A, Daglar K, et al. Balloon tamponade for the management of postpartum uterine hemorrhage. J Perinat Med 2014;42(6):745–53.

20. Tan CH, Tay KH, Sheah K, et al. Perioperative endovascular internal iliac artery occlusion balloon placement in management of placenta accreta. AJR Am J Roentgenol 2007;189:1158–63.

21. Ballas J, Hull AD, Saenz C, et al. Preoperative intravascular balloon catheters and surgical outcomes in pregnancies complicated by placenta accreta: a management paradox. Am J Obstet Gynecol 2012;207(3):216.e1–5.

22. Salim R, Chulski A, Romano S, et al. Precesarean prophylactic balloon catheters for suspected placenta accreta. Obstet Gynecol 2015;126:1022–8.

23. Sovik E, Stokkeland P, Storm BS, et al. The use of aortic occlusion balloon catheter without fluoroscopy for life-threatening post-partum haemorrhage. Acta Anaesthesiol Scand 2012;56:388–93.

24. Walker MG, Allen L, Windrim RC, et al. Multidisciplinary management of invasive placenta previa. J Obstet Gynaecol Can 2013;35(5):417–25.

25. Izbizky G, Meller C, Grasso M, et al. Feasibility and safety of prophylactic uterine artery catheterization and embolization in the management of placenta accreta. J Vasc Interv Radiol 2015;26:162–9.

26. Angstmann T, Gard G, Harrington T, et al. Surgical management of placenta accreta: a cohort seris and suggested approach. Am J Obstet Gynecol 2010;202: 38.e1–9.

27. Eller AG, Bennett MA, Sharshiner M, et al. Maternal morbidity in cases of placenta accreta managed by a multidisciplinary care team compared with standard obstetric care. Obstet Gynecol 2011;117:331–7.

28. Li Q, Yang Z, Mohammed W, et al. Prophylactic uterine artery embolization assisted cesarean section for the prevention of intrapartum hemorrhage in high-risk patients. Cardiovasc Intervent Radiol 2014;37(6):1458–63.

29. Haider AH, Piper LC, Zogg CK, et al. Military-to-civilian translation of battlefield innovations in operative trauma care. Surgery 2015;158(6):1686–95.

30. Gungorduk K, Yildirim G, Asicioglu C, et al. Can intravenous injection of tranexamic acid be used in routine practice with active management of the third stage of labor in vaginal delivery? A randomized controlled study. Am J Perinatol 2013; 30(5):407–13.
31. Ducloy-Bouthors A, Jude B, Duhamel A, et al. High-dose tranexamic acid reduces blood loss in postpartum haemorrhage. Crit Care 2011;15(2):R117.
32. Novikova N, Hofmeyr G, Cluve G. Tranexamic acid for preventing postpartum haemorrhage. Cochrane Database Syst Rev 2015;(6):CD007872.
33. Achneck HE, Sileshi B, Jamiolkowski RJ, et al. A comprehensive review of topical hemostatic agents; efficacy and recommendations for use. Ann Surg 2010;251: 217–28.
34. Schmid BC, Rezniczek GA, Rolf N, et al. Postpartum hemorrhage: use of hemostatic combat gauze. Am J Obstet Gynecol 2012;206(1):e12–3.
35. Mohanan PV, Rathinam K. The teratogenic potential of bone wax extract in rats. Vet Hum Toxicol 1994;36(2):125–7.
36. Lavigne-Lissalde G, Aya AG, Mercier FJ, et al. Recombinant human FVIIa for reducing the need for invasive second-line therapies in severe refractory postpartum hemorrhage: a multicenter, randomized, open controlled trial. J Thromb Haemost 2015;13(4):520–9.
37. Wu S, Kocherginsky M, Hibbard J. Abnormal placentation: twenty-year analysis. Am J Obstet Gynecol 2005;192(5):1458–61.
38. Bailit JL, Grobman WA, Rice MM, et al. Morbidly adherent placenta treatments and outcomes. Obstet Gynecol 2015;125:683–9.
39. Clark SL, Belfort MA, Dildy GA, et al. Maternal death in the 21st century: causes, prevention, and relationship to cesarean delivery. Am J Obstet Gynecol 2008; 199:36.e1–5.
40. Silver RM, Landon MB, Rouse DJ, et al. Maternal morbidity associated with multiple repeat cesarean deliveries. Obstet Gynecol 2006;107:1226–32.
41. Grobman WA, Gersnoviez R, Landon M, et al. Pregnancy outcomes for women with placenta previa in relation to the number of prior cesarean deliveries. Obstet Gynecol 2007;110(6):1249–55.
42. Yin CS. Pregnancy after hysteroscopic endometrial ablation without endometrial preparation: a case of cases and a literature review. Taiwan J Obstet Gynecol 2010;49:311–9.
43. Publications Committee, Society for Maternal-Fetal Medicine, Belfort MA. Placenta accreta. Am J Obstet Gynecol 2010;203(5):430–9.
44. Timor-Tritsch IE, Monteagudo A, Cali G, et al. Cesarean scar pregnancy is a precursor of morbidly adherent placenta. Ultrasound Obstet Gynecol 2014;44: 346–53.
45. Rota MA, Haberman S, Levgur M. Cesarean scar ectopic pregnancies. Obstet Gynecol 2006;107(6):1371–81.
46. Chantraine F, Blacher S, Berndt S, et al. Abnormal vascular architecture at the placental-maternal interface in placenta increta. Am J Obstet Gynecol 2012; 207:188.e1–9.
47. Bowman ZS, Eller A, Kennedy AM, et al. Accuracy of ultrasound for the prediction of placenta accreta. Am J Obstet Gynecol 2014;211(2):177.e1–7.
48. D'Antonio F, Iacovella C, Bhide A. Prenatal identification of invasive placentation using ultrasound: systematic review and meta-analysis. Ultrasound Obstet Gynecol 2013;42:509–17.

49. D'Antonio F, Iacovella C, Palacios J, et al. Prenatal identification of invasive placentation using magnetic resonance imaging: systematic review and metanalysis. Ultrasound Obstet Gynecol 2014;44(1):8–16.

50. Fitzpatrick KE, Sellers S, Spark P, et al. The management and outcomes of placenta accreta, increta, and percreta in the UK: a population-based descriptive study. BJOG 2014;121:62–71.

51. Silver RM, Fox KA, Barton JR, et al. Center of excellence for placenta accreta. Am J Obstet Gynecol 2015;213(6):755–60.

52. Warshak CR, Ramos GA, Eskander R, et al. Effect of predelivery diagnosis in 99 consecutive cases of placenta accreta. Obstet Gynecol 2010;115:65–9.

53. Eller AG, Porter TF, Soisson P, et al. Optimal management strategies for placenta accreta. BJOG 2009;116:648–54.

54. Shamshirsaz AA, Fox KA, Salmanian B, et al. Maternal morbidity in patients with morbidly adherent placenta treated with and without a standardized multidisciplinary approach. Am J Obstet Gynecol 2015;212:218.e1–9.

55. Wright JD, Pri-Paz S, Herzog TJ, et al. Predictors of massive blood loss in women with placenta accreta. Am J Obstet Gynecol 2011;205:38.e1–6.

56. Robinson BK, Grobman WA. Effectiveness of timing strategies for delivery of individuals with placenta previa and accreta. Obsetet Gynecol 2010;116:835–42.

57. Eshkoli T, Weintraub AY, Sergienko R, et al. Placenta accreta: risk factors, perinatal outcomes, and consequences for subsequent births. Am J Obstet Gynecol 2013;208:219.e1–7.

58. Sentilles L, Ambroselli C, Kayem G, et al. Maternal outcome after conservative treatment of placenta accreta. Obstet Gynecol 2010;115:526–34.

59. Schroder L, Potzsch B, Ruhl H, et al. Tranexamic acid for hyperfibrinolytic hemorrhage during conservative management of placenta percreta. Obstet Gynecol 2015;126:1012–5.

60. Smith ES, Gala RB. Successful management of cesarean scar pregnancy complicated by an arteriovenous malformation. Ochsner J 2015;15:268–71.

61. Judy AE, Lyell DJ, Druzin ML, et al. Disseminated intravascular coagulation complicating the conservative management of placena percreta. Obstet Gynecol 2015;126:1016–8.

62. American College of Obstetricians and Gynecologists. Placena accreta. Committee opinion 529. Obstet Gynecol 2012;120:207–11.

63. Smaill FM, Grivell RM. Antibiotic prophylaxis versus no prophylaxis for preventing infection after cesarean section. Cochrane Database Syst Rev 2014;(10):CD007482.

64. Tuuli MG, Liu J, Tout MJ, et al. A randomized trial comparing skin antiseptic agents at cesarean delivery. N Engl J Med 2016;374(7):647–55.

65. Bazer FW, First NL. Pregnancy and parturition. J Anim Sci 1983;57(Suppl 2): 425–60.

66. Palmer SK, Zamudio S, Coffin C, et al. Quantitative estimation of human uterine artery blood flow and pelvic blood flow redistribution in pregnancy. Obstet Gynecol 1992;80(6):1000–6.

67. Rossetti D, Vitale SG, Bogani G, et al. Usefulness of vessel-sealing devices for peripartum hysterectomy: a retrospective cohort study. Updates Surg 2015; 67(3):301–4.

Management Strategies for the Ovaries at the Time of Hysterectomy for Benign Disease

 CrossMark

Catherine A. Matthews, MD, FACOG, FACS

KEYWORDS

- Elective bilateral salpingo-oophorectomy • BSO • Ovarian removal
- Ovarian conservation • Mortality • Cardiovascular disease • Sexual function
- Hip fracture

KEY POINTS

- For premenopausal women with no evidence for a hereditary ovarian or breast cancer syndrome, elective bilateral salpingo-oophorectomy (BSO) should be discouraged based on an increased risk of cardiovascular disease and sexual dysfunction.
- For postmenopausal women, no conclusive evidence for ovarian conservation exists for coronary heart disease prevention, hip fracture prevention, or improved sexual function. Leaving the ovaries in situ increases the risk of incident breast and ovarian cancer and need for subsequent adnexal surgery for benign and malignant disease.
- Opportunistic salpingectomy should be universally encouraged.
- Age 65 is an artificial cutoff value for ovarian removal based on a mathematical decision model and likely has little relevance in clinical practice.

INTRODUCTION

Every woman undergoing hysterectomy for benign disease is faced with the complex and controversial decision of what to do with the ancillary uterine structures, the fallopian tubes, ovaries, and cervix. Many women feel inadequately informed about their treatment options.[1] Gynecologic surgeons will likely play the most influential role in a woman's medical decision-making. Over the past 15 years, a dramatic shift has been observed in national trends of adnexal surgeries at the time of hysterectomy. A recent cross-sectional analysis of all hysterectomies for benign disease performed in the United States reported a 3.6% annual decline in bilateral salpingo-oophorectomy

Department of Obstetrics and Gynecology, Wake Forest University Medical Center, 1 Medical Center Boulevard, Winston Salem, NC 27157, USA
E-mail address: camatthe@wakehealth.edu

Obstet Gynecol Clin N Am 43 (2016) 539–549
http://dx.doi.org/10.1016/j.ogc.2016.04.011
0889-8545/16/$ – see front matter © 2016 Elsevier Inc. All rights reserved.

obgyn.theclinics.com

(BSO) rates from 49.7% in 2001 to 33.4% in 2011.[2] The impetus for this practice change largely hinged on analyses reported from the Nurses' Health Study.[3,4]

Unfortunately, despite more than 600,000 hysterectomies performed annually in the United States, no prospective randomized trials exist to provide the gold-standard evidence on the effects of ovarian conservation versus removal in women deemed average risk for ovarian cancer. Medical counseling and decision making regarding BSO, therefore, is largely based on observational studies or models that are inherently limited by the potential for bias and confounding. As evidenced by the disparate outcomes of a prospective randomized trial on postmenopausal estrogen replacement therapy compared with the multitude of prior epidemiologic studies, we are currently not well equipped with level I evidence to objectively counsel women about this issue.

The principal motivation for elective BSO is a reduction in risk of subsequent ovarian abnormality. Ovarian cancer remains the most lethal gynecologic malignancy with no effective screening method. Despite advances in medical and surgical treatments of this disease, long-term survival remains poor with a 5-year overall survival of 45%.[5] Hysterectomy with BSO has also demonstrated a beneficial effect on total cancer risk, largely driven by a protective effect on incident breast cancer.[6]

The beneficial effects of elective BSO on ovarian and breast cancer, however, must be weighed against the potential negative effects of premature withdrawal of ovarian hormones on cardiovascular disease, hip fracture, sexual function, and overall mortality.[7] Reluctance to prescribe long-term estrogen replacement therapy in the wake of the Women's Health Study has likely also affected the decision to proceed with BSO.[8]

The purpose of this article is to summarize the existing evidence on elective ovarian removal at the time of hysterectomy for benign disease to maximize shared decision making regarding this important topic. The author evaluates the impact of BSO on the specific health issues of total cancer risk, ovarian and breast cancer, heart disease, overall mortality, sexual and cognitive function, and osteoporotic hip fractures. A suggested algorithm for management is provided in **Fig. 1** based on summary recommendations.

ELECTIVE VERSUS RISK-REDUCING BILATERAL SALPINGO-OOPHORECTOMY AND OVARIAN CANCER

In 2012, there were approximately 239,000 new cases of ovarian cancer reported worldwide.[9] When considering the question of elective BSO at the time of routine hysterectomy, it is imperative to correctly identify those women who are indeed "low risk" and have no increased genetic susceptibility for breast or ovarian cancer.[10] Women with a strong family history of breast or ovarian cancer may be carriers of a BRCA1 or BRCA2 germline mutation that accounts for 95% of hereditary ovarian cancer cases. Women with 2 first-degree relatives with either breast or ovarian cancer should be considered as potentially having this autosomal-dominant germline mutation even in the absence of genetic testing.[11]

BRCA1 or BRCA2 germline mutations are associated with a 15% to 60% lifetime risk of developing ovarian cancer compared with only 1.4% in the general population.[12] Women with these mutations should be counseled about risk-reducing BSO as soon as childbearing is complete.[13–15]

Gynecologists are responsible for accurately soliciting a comprehensive family history to detect possible cases of hereditary cancer syndromes. Family history can easily be forgotten when focused on the primary indication for the hysterectomy, such as complicated uterine fibroids. The American Cancer Society estimates that almost 22,000 women will be diagnosed with ovarian cancer in the United States

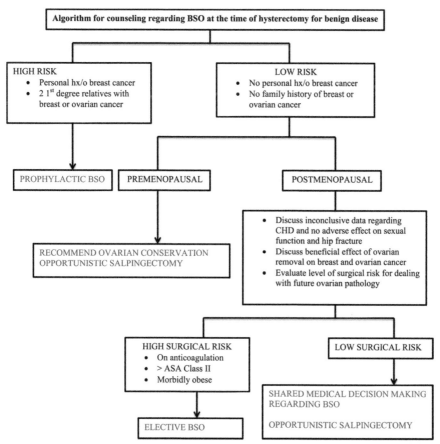

Fig. 1. Algorithm for counseling regarding BSO at the time of hysterectomy for benign disease.

and 14,180 will die of the disease in 2015.[16] Approximately 1000 new cases could be prevented annually if each woman undergoing hysterectomy had an elective BSO.

OPPORTUNISTIC SALPINGECTOMY

The pathogenesis of high-grade serous carcinomas is now thought to originate from precursor lesions in the fallopian tubes rather than the ovarian surface.[17–21] Evidence from molecular and genetic studies supports this new theory that has important implications for pelvic surgeons. The tubes and ovaries have commonly been viewed as a single "adnexal" structure, and discussion has focused on ovarian removal with little consideration given to isolated salpingectomy. Fallopian tubes can be electively removed at the time of hysterectomy to reduce the risk of future ovarian cancer with no deleterious effect on ovarian function, a practice now coined "opportunistic salpingectomy."[22] Although this strategy maximizes residual ovarian function, it does not eliminate the need for subsequent adnexal surgery for pain or other ovarian abnormality. Since 2009, a dramatic increase in concomitant bilateral salpingectomy has been observed.[2]

Despite the absence of prospective evidence that salpingectomy decreases the incidence of ovarian cancer, the 2015 Society of Gynecologic Oncology recommendations for the prevention of ovarian cancer expressly stipulate that salpingectomy should be considered an alternative strategy to other sterilization techniques and performed opportunistically at the time of hysterectomy or other pelvic surgery.[23] The British Columbia Ovarian Cancer Prevention Project estimates that opportunistic salpingectomy could result in up to a 50% reduction in ovarian cancer deaths after 20 years, 20% of which would result from routine bilateral salpingectomy at the time of benign hysterectomy.[24] Even in women with confirmed BRCA mutations, bilateral salpingectomy with delayed oophorectomy has been deemed a cost-effective and acceptable alternative when considering quality-adjusted life experience.[25]

There is evidence of successful dissemination of this information: a recent report that evaluated national trends in adnexal surgeries in the United States demonstrated a 24% increase in the annual rate of bilateral salpingectomy, with almost a quadrupled rate over the 14-year study period.[2] This study was limited in that only inpatient hospital admissions were reviewed. As most benign hysterectomies are now performed on an outpatient basis, it is possible that these results differ.

HYSTERECTOMY WITH AND WITHOUT BILATERAL SALPINGO-OOPHORECTOMY AND INCIDENT CANCER RISK

Two comprehensive analyses of BSO and incident cancer risk have identified a total cancer reduction,[3,6] whereas the Women's Health Initiative (WHI) Observational Study only demonstrated an impact on ovarian cancer risk.[26] In the Nurses' Health Study of 29,380 women over 24 years of follow-up, breast (multivariate hazard ratio [HR] 0.75, 95% confidence interval [CI] 0.68–0.84), ovarian (HR 0.04, 95% CI 0.01–0.09), and total cancers (HR 0.90, 95% CI 0.84–0.96) were reduced in the BSO group. The negative association with total cancers was found despite a reported higher risk of lung cancer in the hysterectomy with BSO group.[3]

Similarly, in a much larger recent study of 66,802 postmenopausal women from the Cancer Prevention Study-II Nutrition Cohort during a mean follow-up of 13.9 years, hysterectomy with BSO performed at any age compared with no hysterectomy was associated with a 10% reduction in all cancers (relative risk [RR] 0.90, 95% CI 0.85–0.96). These results were principally driven by breast cancer in which hysterectomy with BSO performed at any age was associated with a 20% reduction in incidence (RR 0.80, 95% CI 0.73–0.88). The greatest protective effect on breast cancer was observed in women with BSO performed before age 45. Even in women 55 or older, however, there was still a significant decrease in breast cancer incidence with ovarian removal (RR 0.81, 95% CI 0.73–0.98). In this study, when current and former smokers who quit less than 20 years before baseline were excluded, there was no association found between BSO and lung cancer.[6]

Another finding from the Cancer Prevention Cohort study was regarding incident ovarian cancers. Although BSO at any age was strongly associated with a lower risk of ovarian cancer (RR 0.12, 95% CI 0.07–0.21), women who underwent simple hysterectomy at any age actually had a higher risk of ovarian cancer than those who had never had surgery (RR 1.36, 95% CI 1.03–1.78). This risk was highest in women aged 45 to 54 (RR 1.53, 95% CI 1.01–2.33). As these data are based on only 14 women who later developed ovarian cancer, the results should be interpreted with some caution. However, this observation has similarly been shown in other studies.[21,27–29] It is certainly plausible that the primary indication for the hysterectomy itself could bias the rate of incident ovarian cancer. For example, endometrioid ovarian cancer can develop from atypical endometriosis tissue, a common indication for primary hysterectomy. As the Nurses' Health Study only evaluated women undergoing hysterectomy with or without BSO, there was no control referent group in that trial to evaluate the impact of hysterectomy alone on incident ovarian cancer.

The results of these 2 large trials highlight the need to discuss not just incident ovarian cancer but also incident breast cancer when deciding on elective BSO. As the protective effects of BSO on ovarian and breast cancer are observed at any age, careful attention to this issue during counseling is required.

BILATERAL SALPINGO-OOPHORECTOMY AND OVERALL MORTALITY

An analysis of the long-term results of the Nurses' Health Study reported an increased risk of all-cause mortality in women undergoing hysterectomy with BSO before age 50 (HR 1.12, 95% CI 1.03–1.21).[7] In this study of 29,380 women over 24 years of follow-up, they reported 350 (10.9%) deaths from coronary heart disease (CHD), 336 (10.5%) from lung cancer, 219 (6.9%) from stroke, 230 (7.2%) from breast cancer, 37 (1.2%) from ovarian cancer, and 118 (3.7%) from colorectal cancer. The observed increase in all-cause mortality in the BSO group was driven by the increased risk of death from lung cancer (HR 1.31, 95% CI 1.02–1.68) and CHD in women younger than age 45 (HR 1.26, 95% CI 1.04–1.54). As stated previously, the observed association with lung cancer was not observed in the other 2 large observational studies.[6,26]

In contrast, all-cause mortality was not increased in a prospective cohort of 25,448 postmenopausal women aged 50 to 79 years enrolled in the WHI Observational Study.[26] Women with a history of hysterectomy and BSO (n = 14,254) versus hysterectomy with ovarian conservation (n = 11,194) had no difference in incident death from all causes (odds ratio [OR] 0.98, 95% CI 0.87–1.10). Similarly, in a much smaller cohort study of women from Olmsted County, Minnesota overall mortality was not increased in women who underwent BSO compared with referent women. In the subset of women who underwent BSO before the age of 45, however, an observed association with increased mortality was observed.[30]

Before the results of the WHI Observational Study, a Markov decision analysis model was constructed that primarily used data on ovarian cancer, CHD, hip fracture, breast cancer, and stroke that was derived from a single cohort study among premenopausal women who had never used estrogen.[4] This model demonstrated an 8.58% rate of excess mortality when BSO is performed before age 55. The conclusion was made that ovarian conservation until age 65 benefits long-term survival. This study was likely very influential in changing gynecologists' practice patterns regarding elective BSO in postmenopausal women. As new and contrasting information from the WHI observational cohort study and the Cancer Prevention Study-II is now available, this model should be interpreted with caution. These conflicting data demonstrate the vital importance of age stratification when evaluating the impact of BSO on overall mortality and extrapolation of results gleaned from the youngest cohort to all women undergoing BSO is not accurate.

CORONARY HEART DISEASE

The greatest argument against ovarian removal has rested on the assertion that premature ovarian hormone withdrawal results in an increased rate of incident CHD, a disease associated with the greatest risk of overall mortality in women. A comprehensive systemic review of 7 large observational studies published in 2009, however, found that the evidence is inconclusive to determine the overall effect of BSO on risk of CHD.[31]

The proposed mechanism whereby BSO increases CHD risk is inducing premature menopause, a condition associated with a higher risk of death from cardiovascular disease.[32,33] Some observational studies have found an increased rate of fatal and/or nonfatal CHD after BSO,[7,32–35] whereas others have not.[26,31,36–38] These conflicting data may be a result of some studies that are limited by small sample size, lack of multivariate analyses, comparison groups of women who did not undergo hysterectomy, and inattention to use of hormone replacement therapy among participants.

In the WHI Prospective Observational Study, women with a history of hysterectomy and BSO (n = 14,254) or hysterectomy with ovarian conservation (n = 11,194), the BSO group did not demonstrate an increased risk of fatal and nonfatal CHD (HR 1.00, 95% CI, 0.85–1.18) or total cardiovascular disease (HR 0.99, 95% CI 0.91–1.09).[26] These negative findings were similar for the BSO group regardless of age at hysterectomy. It is important to note that the vast majority of women (79%) reported current, or past use, of hormone replacement therapy, a finding which could have attenuated CHD risk in the younger women.

In contrast, the Nurses' Health Study reported a significant association between BSO and CHD, but these results require careful inspection.[3] The study authors reported that in the overall cohort, BSO was associated with a significantly increased risk of fatal and nonfatal heart disease. When the risk of incident events is evaluated by age, however, one notes that the significant association between CHD and BSO was derived solely from the cohort of women younger than 45 years. Their multivariate HR was 1.34 (95% CI 1.13–1.60). In contrast, women aged 45 to 54 (HR 1.08 [0.86–1.35]) and 55 and older (HR 0.99 [0.64–1.54]) had no significant association observed. When the cohort was evaluated collectively, a small increased risk, driven by the findings in the young cohort, was observed (HR 1.17 [1.02–1.35]).

The importance of understanding this variable but profound effect of BSO on CHD risk at different ages is best illustrated by the commonly cited results of a Markov decision analysis, a mathematical model designed to resolve the optimal age for BSO.[4] It was this previously referenced model that cited 65 as the "rational" cutoff age for ovarian removal. In the model, a hypothetical cohort of patients was followed over time, and disease incidence was calculated based on estimated probabilities from the medical literature. The investigators acknowledged that their estimates of survival were very sensitive to changes in the RR of CHD. In the base case, they assigned a CHD RR of 2.2 (95% CI 1.2–4.2) for women after BSO up to age 55 years when estrogen was not used, a value obtained from an earlier analysis of participants in the Nurses Health Study.[32] Based on this RR, the model calculated that ovarian conservation without estrogen therapy reduces the proportion of women dying from CHD in the base case from 15.95% to 7.57%. These reductions are in vast excess of women who die from ovarian cancer, and therefore, ovarian conservation was endorsed.

The primary fault of this Markov model lies in the erroneous estimate of CHD risk that was derived only from women under age 45 but was then applied to the overall population. Furthermore, the assigned CHD RR of 2.2 is double the observed HR of women in this same age group reported from the Nurses' Health Study in 2009 (HR 1.34 [95% CI 1.13–1.60]).[3] This model, therefore, grossly overestimated the negative effect of ovarian removal based on an erroneously high rate of CHD.

In 2013, a further analysis of updated data from the same Nurses' Health Study cohort was published.[7] Overall, 16.8% of women with hysterectomy and BSO died of all causes compared with 13.3% who had ovarian conservation. Elective BSO in women aged younger than 50 who never used estrogen therapy was again associated with increased cardiovascular mortality (HR 1.29 [1.01–1.64]). In those aged 50 to 59 years, however, no significant association was observed (HR 0.78 [0.42–1.46]).

From these data, it is apparent that elective BSO performed in women under the age of 50 who do not take hormone therapy is associated with a higher rate of CHD and should be discouraged. In women over the age of 50, however, BSO has not been associated with increased risk of incident CHD and should not be used as the principal argument for ovarian conservation.

SEXUAL FUNCTION

Premenopausal women who undergo BSO experience an abrupt decline in circulating estrogen and testosterone levels, which can result in vaginal dryness, dyspareunia, and loss of libido. One study reported a higher frequency of hypoactive sexual desire disorder in women younger than 50 with BSO compared with those with ovarian conservation,[39] whereas another found no difference in any measure of health-related quality of life or sexual functioning at 2 years postoperatively.[40] Sexual function, however, can be difficult to assess in an unbiased fashion in observational studies due to the interaction of other nonhormonal variables such as relationship status and body image. For example, in younger women undergoing risk-reducing BSO, relationship satisfaction was associated with a significantly lower rate of sexual dysfunction, and there was no correlation between serum testosterone and sexual satisfaction.[41]

Young women undergoing risk-reducing BSO, in which deprivation of estrogen and testosterone occurs acutely, have reported a high rate of female sexual dysfunction (74%), hypoactive sexual desire disorder (73%), lubrication difficulty (44%) dyspareunia (28%), and orgasmic dysfunction (25%).[41] In premenopausal women, some of the symptoms of sexual dysfunction can be reversed with hormone replacement therapy.[42] Although estrogen supplementation is easily achieved with oral or transdermal formulations, testosterone supplementation is more difficult because of poor oral bioavailability.[43]

Postmenopausal women who undergo BSO also experience a decline in circulating testosterone concentrations because the ovarian stroma continues to be biologically active following menopause.[44] The overall effect of BSO on sexual function in postmenopausal women, however, appears to be minimal. From a cross-sectional analysis of 1352 postmenopausal, community-dwelling women designed to investigate sexuality in older adults, women with previous BSO (n = 356) were compared with women with retained ovaries (n = 996). Despite a decline in sexual activity, frequency, and attitude among the cohort with age, no significant difference in the report of sexual ideation was found in multivariate analysis in women with BSO (54.5%) versus ovarian conservation (49.9%). Furthermore, reports of sexual problems such as lack of interest, vaginal lubrication, anorgasmia, pain, and lack of pleasure were not different between the 2 groups.[45]

OSTEOPOROTIC HIP FRACTURES

Estrogen deprivation states are well known to cause osteoporotic hip fractures. The data from large observational studies regarding the effect of BSO on hip fracture risk, however, demonstrate no adverse effect. In the prospective observational study of almost 30,000 women in the Nurses' Health Study, no difference in hip fractures existed in either premenopausal or postmenopausal women who had BSO.[3] Similarly, in a study of 6295 women participating in the Study of Osteoporotic Fractures, postmenopausal BSO was not associated with an increased risk of either hip or vertebral fractures despite a lower serum testosterone concentration in the BSO group.[46] The

WHI Observational Study also showed no increased risk of fracture in women with BSO (HR 0.83 [95% CI 0.63–1.10]).[26] Only 1 small study of 340 postmenopausal women from Olmsted County, Minnesota reported a significant increase in the risk of any osteoporotic fracture.[47] It is possible that relative to other risk factors for osteoporosis, BSO plays a very minor role, and thus, no association has been demonstrated from 3 large studies.

SUBSEQUENT ADNEXAL SURGERY

Up to 9% of women require future surgery if BSO is not performed at the time of hysterectomy,[48–51] a risk that is approximately 2% higher than those without simple hysterectomy. In a population-based study of 4931 women in Olmsted County, Minnesota who underwent hysterectomy alone for benign indications (case group) versus a similar referent group without hysterectomy, the respective cumulative incidences of subsequent oophorectomy were 3.5%, 6.2%, and 9.2% among cases and 1.9%, 4.8%, and 7.3% among controls at 10, 20, and 30 years after hysterectomy. The overall risk of subsequent oophorectomy among case group participants was significantly higher than among referent group participants (HR 1.20, 95% CI 1.02–1.42; $P = .03$). Furthermore, among case group participants, the risk of subsequent oophorectomy was significantly higher (HR 2.15, 95% CI 1.51–3.07; $P<.001$) in women who had both ovaries preserved compared with those who initially had one ovary preserved.[51] In another cohort study of 2561 women with retained ovaries, the most common reasons for subsequent oophorectomy were pain (71%) and the presence of an asymptomatic adnexal mass (25%).[50] Careful consideration for elective BSO should be made for women who are at higher surgical risk if future operative intervention is required, such as those on anticoagulation therapy, known severe adhesive disease, or morbid obesity.

BILATERAL SALPINGO-OOPHORECTOMY AND ROUTE OF HYSTERECTOMY

In theory, the surgical route of hysterectomy should have little bearing on counseling regarding ovarian removal or conservation. Vaginal hysterectomy, however, has been associated with significantly lower rates of concomitant BSO.[52] In a cross-sectional analysis of 461,321 hysterectomies performed in the United States, women undergoing laparoscopic hysterectomy were 8 times more likely, and those undergoing abdominal hysterectomy 12 times more likely to have BSO compared with a vaginal approach.[53] Another large cross-sectional study demonstrated dramatic differences in BSO rates between abdominal (54%), laparoscopic (50%), and vaginal (17%) routes of hysterectomy.[54] Although a vaginal approach may limit visualization of the adnexae, surgical techniques for vaginal ovarian removal are well described and should be mastered by anyone offering this route of surgery for hysterectomy.[55]

SUMMARY

The pendulum has likely swung too far in favor of ovarian conservation for all women under 65 undergoing hysterectomy for benign disease. For premenopausal women with no evidence for a hereditary ovarian or breast cancer syndrome, elective BSO should be discouraged based on an increased risk of cardiovascular disease and sexual dysfunction. Opportunistic salpingectomy, however, should be universally encouraged. For postmenopausal women, no conclusive evidence for ovarian conservation exists for overall mortality, CHD prevention, hip fracture prevention, or improved sexual function. This practice does, however, have a proven negative effect on incident ovarian and breast cancer. Leaving the ovaries in situ may increase the risk of subsequent adnexal surgery and nonserous ovarian cancer. Age 65 is an artificial cutoff value for ovarian removal based on a mathematical decision model and likely has little relevance in clinical practice. Based on the best available evidence from the current literature, careful consideration for elective ovarian removal should be advocated for all postmenopausal women undergoing hysterectomy for benign disease.

REFERENCES

1. Bhavnani V, Clarke A. Women awaiting hysterectomy: a qualitative study of issues involved in decisions about oophorectomy. BJOG 2003;110(2):168–74.
2. Mikhail E, Salemi JL, Mogos MF, et al. National trends of adnexal surgeries at the time of hysterectomy for benign indication, United States, 1998-2011. Am J Obstet Gynecol 2015;213(5):713.e1–13.
3. Parker WH, Broder MS, Chang E, et al. Ovarian conservation at the time of hysterectomy and long-term health outcomes in the Nurses' Health Study. Obstet Gynecol 2009;113(5):1027–37.
4. Parker WH, Broder MS, Liu Z, et al. Ovarian conservation at the time of hysterectomy for benign disease. Obstet Gynecol 2005;106(2):219–26.
5. Tanner EJ, Long KC, Visvanathan K, et al. Prophylactic salpingectomy in premenopausal women at low risk for ovarian cancer: risk-reducing or risky? Fertil Steril 2013;100(6):1530–1.
6. Gaudet MM, Gapstur SM, Sun J, et al. Oophorectomy and hysterectomy and cancer incidence in the Cancer Prevention Study-II Nutrition Cohort. Obstet Gynecol 2014;123(6):1247–55.
7. Parker WH, Feskanich D, Broder MS, et al. Long-term mortality associated with oophorectomy compared with ovarian conservation in the Nurses' Health Study. Obstet Gynecol 2013;121(4):709–16.
8. Asante A, Whiteman MK, Kulkarni A, et al. Elective oophorectomy in the United States: trends and in-hospital complications, 1998-2006. Obstet Gynecol 2010;116(5):1088–95.
9. World Cancer Research Fund/American Institute for Cancer Research Continuous Update Project Report. Food, Nutrition, Physical Activity, and the Prevention of Ovarian Cancer 2014. Available at: http://www.dietandcancerreport.org/cup/cup_resources.php. Accessed February 1, 2016.
10. Berek JS, Chalas E, Edelson M, et al. Prophylactic and risk-reducing bilateral salpingo-oophorectomy: recommendations based on risk of ovarian cancer. Obstet Gynecol 2010;116(3):733–43.
11. Hogg R, Friedlander M. Biology of epithelial ovarian cancer: implications for screening women at high genetic risk. J Clin Oncol 2004;22(7):1315–27.
12. ACOG. ACOG practice bulletin no. 89. Elective and risk-reducing salpingo-oophorectomy. Obstet Gynecol 2008;111(1):231–41.
13. Rebbeck TR, Kauff ND, Domchek SM. Meta-analysis of risk reduction estimates associated with risk-reducing salpingo-oophorectomy in BRCA1 or BRCA2 mutation carriers. J Natl Cancer Inst 2009;101(2):80–7.
14. Boyd J. Molecular genetics of hereditary ovarian cancer. Oncology (Williston Park) 1998;12(3):399–406.
15. Kauff ND, Satagopan JM, Robson ME, et al. Risk-reducing salpingo-oophorectomy in women with a BRCA1 or BRCA2 mutation. N Engl J Med 2002;346(21):1609–15.

16. Cancer Facts and Figures 2015. Available at: http://www.cancer.org/acs/groups/content/@editorial/documents/document/acspc-044552.pdf. Accessed February 1, 2016.

17. Carlson J, Roh MH, Chang MC, et al. Recent advances in the understanding of the pathogenesis of serous carcinoma: the concept of low- and high-grade disease and the role of the fallopian tube. Diagn Histopathol (Oxf) 2008;14(8):352–65.

18. Carlson JW, Miron A, Jarboe EA, et al. Serous tubal intraepithelial carcinoma: its potential role in primary peritoneal serous carcinoma and serous cancer prevention. J Clin Oncol 2008;26(25):4160–5.

19. Crum CP, Drapkin R, Kindelberger D, et al. Lessons from BRCA: the tubal fimbria emerges as an origin for pelvic serous cancer. Clin Med Res 2007;5(1):35–44.

20. Przybycin CG, Kurman RJ, Ronnett BM, et al. Are all pelvic (nonuterine) serous carcinomas of tubal origin? Am J Surg Pathol 2010;34(10):1407–16.

21. Nagle CM, Olsen CM, Webb PM, et al. Endometrioid and clear cell ovarian cancers: a comparative analysis of risk factors. Eur J Cancer 2008;44(16):2477–84.

22. Morelli M, Venturella R, Zullo F. Risk-reducing salpingectomy as a new and safe strategy to prevent ovarian cancer. Am J Obstet Gynecol 2013;209(4):395–6.

23. Walker JL, Powell CB, Chen LM, et al. Society of gynecologic oncology recommendations for the prevention of ovarian cancer. Cancer 2015;121(13):2108–20.

24. Morelli M, Venturella R, Mocciaro R, et al. Prophylactic salpingectomy in premenopausal low-risk women for ovarian cancer: primum non nocere. Gynecol Oncol 2013;129(3):448–51.

25. Kwon JS, Tinker A, Pansegrau G, et al. Prophylactic salpingectomy and delayed oophorectomy as an alternative for BRCA mutation carriers. Obstet Gynecol 2013;121(1):14–24.

26. Jacoby VL, Grady D, Wactawski-Wende J, et al. Oophorectomy vs ovarian conservation with hysterectomy: cardiovascular disease, hip fracture, and cancer in the Women's Health Initiative Observational Study. Arch Intern Med 2011;171(8):760–8.

27. Jordan SJ, Nagle CM, Coory MD, et al. Has the association between hysterectomy and ovarian cancer changed over time? A systematic review and meta-analysis. Eur J Cancer 2013;49(17):3638–47.

28. Ness RB, Dodge RC, Edwards RP, et al. Contraception methods, beyond oral contraceptives and tubal ligation, and risk of ovarian cancer. Ann Epidemiol 2011;21(3):188–96.

29. Jordan SJ, Green AC, Whiteman DC, et al. Serous ovarian, fallopian tube and primary peritoneal cancers: a comparative epidemiological analysis. Int J Cancer 2008;122(7):1598–603.

30. Rocca WA, Grossardt BR, de Andrade M, et al. Survival patterns after oophorectomy in premenopausal women: a population-based cohort study. Lancet Oncol 2006;7(10):821–8.

31. Jacoby VL, Grady D, Sawaya GF. Oophorectomy as a risk factor for coronary heart disease. Am J Obstet Gynecol 2009;200(2):140.e1–9.

32. Colditz GA, Willett WC, Stampfer MJ, et al. Menopause and the risk of coronary heart disease in women. N Engl J Med 1987;316(18):1105–10.

33. Gordon T, Kannel WB, Hjortland MC, et al. Menopause and coronary heart disease. The Framingham Study. Ann Intern Med 1978;89(2):157–61.

34. Howard BV, Kuller L, Langer R, et al. Risk of cardiovascular disease by hysterectomy status, with and without oophorectomy: the Women's Health Initiative Observational Study. Circulation 2005;111(12):1462–70.

35. Svanberg L. Effects of estrogen deficiency in women castrated when young. Acta Obstet Gynecol Scand Suppl 1981;106:11–5.
36. Luoto R, Kaprio J, Reunanen A, et al. Cardiovascular morbidity in relation to ovarian function after hysterectomy. Obstet Gynecol 1995;85(4):515–22.
37. Palmer JR, Rosenberg L, Shapiro S. Reproductive factors and risk of myocardial infarction. Am J Epidemiol 1992;136(4):408–16.
38. Ritterband AB, Jaffe IA, Densen PM, et al. Gonadal function and the development of coronary heart disease. Circulation 1963;27:237–51.
39. Leiblum SR, Koochaki PE, Rodenberg CA, et al. Hypoactive sexual desire disorder in postmenopausal women: US results from the Women's International Study of Health and Sexuality (WISHeS). Menopause 2006;13(1):46–56.
40. Teplin V, Vittinghoff E, Lin F, et al. Oophorectomy in premenopausal women: health-related quality of life and sexual functioning. Obstet Gynecol 2007;109(2 Pt 1):347–54.
41. Tucker PE, Bulsara MK, Salfinger SG, et al. Prevalence of sexual dysfunction after risk-reducing salpingo-oophorectomy. Gynecol Oncol 2016;140(1):95–100.
42. Madalinska JB, Hollenstein J, Bleiker E, et al. Quality-of-life effects of prophylactic salpingo-oophorectomy versus gynecologic screening among women at increased risk of hereditary ovarian cancer. J Clin Oncol 2005;23(28):6890–8.
43. Shifren JL, Braunstein GD, Simon JA, et al. Transdermal testosterone treatment in women with impaired sexual function after oophorectomy. N Engl J Med 2000;343(10):682–8.
44. Judd HL, Lucas WE, Yen SS. Effect of oophorectomy on circulating testosterone and androstenedione levels in patients with endometrial cancer. Am J Obstet Gynecol 1974;118(6):793–8.
45. Erekson EA, Martin DK, Zhu K, et al. Sexual function in older women after oophorectomy. Obstet Gynecol 2012;120(4):833–42.
46. Antoniucci DM, Sellmeyer DE, Cauley JA, et al. Postmenopausal bilateral oophorectomy is not associated with increased fracture risk in older women. J Bone Miner Res 2005;20(5):741–7.
47. Melton LJ 3rd, Crowson CS, Malkasian GD, et al. Fracture risk following bilateral oophorectomy. J Clin Epidemiol 1996;49(10):1111–5.
48. Dekel A, Efrat Z, Orvieto R, et al. The residual ovary syndrome: a 20-year experience. Eur J Obstet Gynecol Reprod Biol 1996;68(1–2):159–64.
49. Zalel Y, Lurie S, Beyth Y, et al. Is it necessary to perform a prophylactic oophorectomy during hysterectomy? Eur J Obstet Gynecol Reprod Biol 1997;73(1):67–70.
50. Holub Z, Jandourek M, Jabor A, et al. Does hysterectomy without salpingo-oophorectomy influence the reoperation rate for adnexal pathology? A retrospective study. Clin Exp Obstet Gynecol 2000;27(2):109–12.
51. Casiano ER, Trabuco EC, Bharucha AE, et al. Risk of oophorectomy after hysterectomy. Obstet Gynecol 2013;121(5):1069–74.
52. Gross CP, Nicholson W, Powe NR. Factors affecting prophylactic oophorectomy in postmenopausal women. Obstet Gynecol 1999;94(6):962–8.
53. Jacoby VL, Vittinghoff E, Nakagawa S, et al. Factors associated with undergoing bilateral salpingo-oophorectomy at the time of hysterectomy for benign conditions. Obstet Gynecol 2009;113(6):1259–67.
54. Jacoby VL, Autry A, Jacobson G, et al. Nationwide use of laparoscopic hysterectomy compared with abdominal and vaginal approaches. Obstet Gynecol 2009;114(5):1041–8.
55. Falcone T, Walters MD. Hysterectomy for benign disease. Obstet Gynecol 2008;111(3):753–67.

Enhanced Recovery Pathway in Gynecologic Surgery

Improving Outcomes Through Evidence-Based Medicine

Eleftheria Kalogera, MD[a], Sean C. Dowdy, MD[b],*

KEYWORDS

- Enhanced recovery • Perioperative care • Gynecologic surgery • Benign
- Abdominal hysterectomy • Vaginal hysterectomy • Laparoscopic hysterectomy

KEY POINTS

- Enhanced recovery after surgery (ERAS) is an evidence-based approach to perioperative care shown to hasten recovery and attenuate the stress response to surgery.
- ERAS principles include preoperative patient education; avoidance of prolonged preoperative fasting, and bowel preparation; multimodal analgesia; perioperative euvolemia; intraoperative normothermia; early oral intake; early mobilization.
- ERAS is associated with earlier return of gastrointestinal function, reduced opioid use, shorter length of stay, stable complication and readmission rates, and substantial cost reductions.

INTRODUCTION

In recent years, a paradigm shift from traditional perioperative care models to the "Enhanced Recovery Pathway (ERP)" or "Enhanced Recovery After Surgery (ERAS)" has taken place across a wide range of surgical specialties including gynecologic surgery. These programs, also known as "Fast-Track Surgery (FTS)," are not new; they were first introduced in the 1990s by European surgeons and anesthesiologists, pioneered in particular by Kehlet, and challenged the efficacy of longstanding, non-evidence-based practices of perioperative care.[1] Surgical stress forces the body

Disclosure: There are no conflicts of interest for this article.
[a] Department of Obstetrics and Gynecology, Mayo Clinic, 200 1st Street Southwest, Rochester, MN 55905, USA; [b] Division of Gynecologic Surgery, Mayo Clinic, 200 1st Street Southwest, Rochester, MN 55905, USA
* Corresponding author.
E-mail address: dowdy.sean@mayo.edu

Obstet Gynecol Clin N Am 43 (2016) 551–573
http://dx.doi.org/10.1016/j.ogc.2016.04.006
0889-8545/16/$ – see front matter © 2016 Elsevier Inc. All rights reserved.

into a highly catabolic state with increased cardiac demands, relative tissue hypoxia, increased insulin resistance, impaired coagulation profile, and altered pulmonary and gastrointestinal functions.[2] The body's response to surgical stress results in organ dysfunction, increased morbidity, and, ultimately, delayed convalescence.[3,4] The ERAS programs aim to maintain normal physiology perioperatively and optimize patient outcomes by introducing interventions that have been proven to either decrease surgical stress or help the body mitigate the negative consequences associated with it.

The ERAS pathways do not base their success on the incorporation of a single intervention into clinical practice but rather represent a multimodal approach to perioperative recovery. The main ERAS elements differ drastically from traditional care and can be divided into preoperative, intraoperative, and postoperative interventions. These elements include preoperative patient education and counseling, minimizing preoperative fasting, avoiding bowel preparation and dehydration, preemptive analgesia, nausea and vomiting prophylaxis, tailored anesthesia with a focus on short-acting anesthetics and regional anesthesia, goal-oriented fluid management to achieve perioperative euvolemia, intraoperative normothermia, no routine use of drain and nasogastric tubes (NGTs), early oral intake, early mobilization, early catheter removal, a preference for nonopioid analgesics, and preemptive use of laxatives. Importantly, the successful implementation of these programs is based on the collaborative work of a multidisciplinary team consisting of surgeons, anesthesiologists, nursing staff, and pharmacists, as well as the active engagement of the patient in enhancing their recovery.

ERAS pathways were initially introduced in colorectal surgery. They have since been successfully implemented in many surgical specialties, including cardiac, thoracic, vascular surgery, urology, and orthopedics. A growing body of evidence suggests that it is both a safe and effective perioperative care approach allowing for shorter length of hospital stay, decreased morbidity, and significant cost reduction without increasing postoperative complication and readmission rates while maintaining high patient satisfaction.[5–11] Notably, a collaborative initiative, called the Enhanced Recovery Partnership Programme, was established in England in 2009 aiming toward the widespread adoption of ERAS in 4 major specialties (colorectal, urology, gynecology, and musculoskeletal).[12,13] Although initially slow, several studies have surfaced over the past few years reporting the successful implementation of this multimodal approach in the perioperative care of the gynecologic surgical patient.

BASIC CONCEPTS OF ENHANCED RECOVERY AFTER SURGERY PATHWAYS
Preoperative

Patient counseling and education
Successful implementation of ERAS pathways to enhance postoperative recovery requires active engagement of all involved parties with the patient playing a central role. Patient counseling should start as early as the initial consult visit and include explaining the rationale behind the ERAS pathway in order to engage the patients in their recovery. In the outpatient setting, providers and nursing staff should identify patient expectations for the hospitalization and educate patients on early mobilization, early postoperative feeding, postoperative pain goals and pain management, and duration of hospitalization. It is helpful for the patients to be given educational materials to take home because this allows patients to familiarize themselves with these concepts. Patient education has been shown to be associated with improved outcomes, including decreased postoperative complications, superior pain control, and shorter recovery

time.[14,15] In order to achieve the goal of an earlier discharge compared with prior practice, early discussion about anticipated hospital length of stay (LOS) and discharge criteria is critical.[16]

Preoperative diet

The rule of NPO (nothing by mouth) at midnight was arbitrarily adopted in an effort to prevent aspiration of gastric contents during anesthesia. However, prolonged fasting is associated with several untoward effects, including patient discomfort, dehydration, caloric restriction, and metabolic changes counter to healing at a time when the body is expected to enter a state of increased metabolic demands. Specifically, a 12-hour period of fasting shifts the body into the metabolic state of starvation; this results in depletion of the liver glycogen stores, a readily available energy source typically mobilized to cover high-energy demands similar to the demands during the immediate postoperative period. These metabolic changes have been shown to adversely affect perioperative outcomes.[17] Fasting has also been associated with impairment of glucose metabolism and an increase in insulin resistance.[18,19] A recent *Cochrane Review* helped shed light on the safety, or lack thereof, of the prolonged fasting: the NPO at midnight rule was not found to be superior to shorter fluid fasting in terms of decreasing the risk of aspiration, regurgitation, or associated morbidity. Interestingly, lower gastric volumes were observed in patients who were allowed to drink water preoperatively.[20] The American Society of Anesthesiology thus recommends fasting from intake of a light meal at least 6 hours and from intake of clear liquids at least 2 hours before elective procedures that require general or regional anesthesia, or sedation/analgesia.[21] Interestingly, ERAS pathways argue in favor of preoperative use of carbohydrate-loading drinks because they are thought to mitigate preoperative caloric restriction, improve insulin resistance,[22] and lead to shorter hospital LOS.[23,24]

Avoiding mechanical bowel preparation

The use of mechanical and antibiotic bowel preparation in abdominal surgery including gynecologic surgery, especially in anticipation of bowel resection, was thought to help decrease the risk of anastomotic leak and prevent perioperative infectious morbidity.[25] The need for bowel preparation has been brought into question especially considering the negative effects associated with their use, such as patient dissatisfaction, dehydration, electrolyte disturbances, need for prolonged fasting, or even a delay in return of bowel function.[26,27] In 2011, a *Cochrane Review* that included 18 randomized controlled trials (RCTs) on the use of mechanical bowel preparation in patients undergoing elective colorectal surgery including rectal surgery concluded that there is no evidence that these patients benefit from mechanical bowel preparation or rectal enemas. The same conclusions were reached in a recent meta-analysis of 5 RCTs focused on gynecologic surgery.[26] Importantly, the investigators of the *Cochrane Review* noted that more data are required in order to guide the use of bowel preparation in elective rectal resections below the peritoneal verge. In light of the lack of conclusive data, the authors of the current review chose to use rectal enemas when anticipating bowel resection especially low anterior resection. Recent data show that oral antibiotic bowel preparation may decrease infection rates in colorectal surgery,[28,29] but high-quality evidence supporting their use in gynecology is lacking. Finally, routine use of mechanical bowel preparation is not recommended in laparoscopic or robotic gynecologic surgery because it offers no benefit with regard to intraoperative visualization or bowel handing.[26,30]

Preemptive analgesia

In ERAS pathways, pain management begins before incision. This theory is based on the concept of preemptive analgesia, in which pain medications block activation of pain receptors before they are activated by the presence of noxious stimuli, resulting in superior pain control and a decrease in pain medication requirements. A multimodal approach incorporating the preoperative use of Gabapentin, oral or intravenous (IV) cyclo-oxygenase (COX) -2 inhibitors (celecoxib or parecoxib), and oral or IV paracetamol, has been associated with decreased use of opioids postoperatively[31–35] and is thus typically used in ERAS protocols.

Intraoperative

Anesthesia

Advances in anesthetic medications and expansion of ambulatory care have allowed application of some of the principles from ambulatory surgery to major surgery, in order to attenuate negative effects of surgical stress and pain, decrease anesthetic-related side effects, and hasten recovery. Short-acting volatile anesthetics or continuous infusion of propofol is recommended to allow rapid surfacing from anesthesia. Rapid awakening is reliably accomplished when these techniques are combined intraoperatively with short-acting opioid analgesics. Total IV anesthesia with propofol has been associated with fewer postoperative side effects and, specifically, a decrease in postoperative nausea and vomiting (PONV).[36–38] The latter is particularly important as both gynecologic surgery as well as minimally invasive surgery have been found to be independent predictors of PONV.[39] Furthermore, regional anesthesia with or without concomitant general anesthesia has been associated with rapid awakening, decreased PONV, and decreased systemic opioid requirements.[40–42]

Maintaining normothermia

Intraoperative body core temperature less than 36°C has been associated with adverse intraoperative and postoperative outcomes, including coagulopathy with increased risk of bleeding, impaired drug metabolism, impaired oxygen transportation and increased peripheral oxygen consumption, cardiac morbidity, and infectious wound morbidity.[43–45] Active warming techniques are used in ERAS pathways. These interventions typically start with prewarming the patient in the preoperative unit in order to minimize the initial drop in core temperature at induction.[46] They are continued throughout surgery and should be extended through the recovery period in the post-anesthesia care unit. Intraoperative use of forced-air blankets, heating mattress pads, circulating-water garments, and IV fluid warming have all been proven effective in preventing hypothermia.[47,48] Continuous intraoperative core body temperature monitoring is critical to guide management of these devices/techniques and to prevent extreme body temperatures, including hypothermia as well as hyperthermia.

Avoiding intraoperative fluid overload

Maintaining euvolemia is a sentinel principle in ERAS pathways. The philosophy of intraoperative fluid management has shifted significantly over the past few decades from liberal fluid administration to restrictive approaches, both of which have been criticized for increasing morbidity and mortality. Fluid overload may lead to electrolyte abnormalities, peripheral soft tissue edema impairing mobility, small bowel edema contributing to delayed return of bowel function, and pulmonary congestion leading to increased pulmonary morbidity. Hypovolemia, in turn, may result in decreased cardiac output affecting oxygen delivery to tissues and thus leading to organ damage. Fluid regimens aiming at negative fluid balance have failed to improve clinical outcomes or shorten hospital LOS compared with traditional fluid regimens.[49] In contrast, perioperative fluid restriction with a goal of euvolemia has been proven superior to the traditional liberal fluid approach. Nisanevich and colleagues[50] observed that intraoperative use of restrictive fluid management resulted in fewer postoperative complications (17% vs 31%, $P<.05$), earlier time to flatus (3 vs 4 days, $P<.001$), earlier bowel movement (4 vs 6 days, $P<.001$), and shorter hospital LOS (8 vs 9 days, $P = .01$) compared with liberal fluid management. Notably, both groups received similar volume of fluids postoperatively. Other investigators have also concluded that perioperative restrictive fluid regimens decrease morbidity.[51,52] A recent meta-analysis of 9 RCTs of nearly 1000 patients corroborates this finding (odds ratio 0.41; $P = .005$).[53] Lobo and colleagues[54] noted that positive fluid balance sufficient to cause as little as 3-kg weight gain postoperatively delays bowel function recovery and prolongs hospital LOS in patients undergoing elective colorectal surgery.

In order to achieve euvolemia intraoperatively within the context of an ERAS protocol, emphasis is placed in minimizing crystalloid and increasing colloid use. If a patient is hypotensive but, at the same time, is thought to be euvolemic (ie, following epidural anesthesia), vasopressor use over liberal crystalloid administration is encouraged. Toward this goal of improved intraoperative fluid management, some ERAS protocols have started to slowly adopt goal-directed therapy. This term is used to describe the use of hemodynamic parameters such as stroke volume, cardiac output, peripheral vascular resistance, or similar parameters to guide IV fluid and inotropic therapy. Data from patients undergoing major abdominal surgery have demonstrated that goal-directed therapy can improve patient outcomes by reducing postoperative complications, expediting return of bowel function, decreasing PONV, reducing intensive care unit admissions, and shortening hospital LOS.[55]

Prevention of postoperative nausea and vomiting

Female gender, gynecologic surgery, and minimally invasive surgery are all well-recognized risk factors for PONV.[39,56] These risk factors may explain at least partially the high prevalence of PONV among women undergoing gynecologic surgery. Rates of PONV in this population are reported as high as 80% and 30%, respectively.[56] PONV contributes to increased patient dissatisfaction, prolonged hospital LOS, and unplanned readmissions. ERAS pathways have thus adopted an aggressive multimodal approach toward preemptive treatment of PONV, which includes intraoperative use of at least 2 agents from different classes of antiemetics.[39,56,57] These classes of antiemetic medication include 5HT3 antagonists, NK-1 antagonists, corticosteroids, antihistamines, anticholinergics, butyrophenones, and phenothiazines.[56,58] Additional strategies to decrease PONV include use of propofol infusion instead of volatile anesthetics or nitrous oxide as well as reduction of opioid use.[39,56] Regional analgesia, although shown to decrease opioid use, did not result in decreased PONV.[59] Patients at high risk for PONV may benefit from application of transdermal scopolamine if applied within 2 hours before anesthesia and surgery.[60]

Avoiding nasogastric tubes

ERAS protocols support limited use of drains, tubes, and catheters and, if needed, their use should be limited to the shortest duration necessary. Traditional perioperative management of surgical patients undergoing abdominal surgery mandated the presence of a NGT until there was evidence of return of bowel function by the presence of either flatus or bowel movement. However, an overwhelming body of evidence now argues against this practice. A Cochrane Review of 33 RCTs found that selective or no NGT use was associated with earlier return of bowel function ($P<.001$), decrease in pulmonary complications ($P = .01$), a trend toward shorter LOS, and no change in anastomotic leak rates or other postoperative complications compared with routine NGT use. The investigators of that review concluded that routine NGT use should be abandoned.[61] Moreover, routine NGT use has been associated with higher rates of postoperative pneumonia, atelectasis, and fever.[62] Cutillo and colleagues[63] compared early oral feeding to NGT decompression combined with feeding at the first passage of flatus in patients undergoing surgery for gynecologic malignancies. They noted that early oral feeding was associated with earlier resolution of ileus, more rapid return to regular diet, no difference in rates of PONV, earlier time to first bowel movement, and shorter LOS. The ERAS Society recommends against routine NGT placement in both benign gynecologic surgery and gynecologic oncology.[64]

Limiting prophylactic peritoneal drains

Although prophylactic use of drains was initially introduced in order to control postoperative fluid collections and aid in early detection of surgical bleeding or anastomotic leak, data have failed to support their effectiveness.[65,66] Most of this data are derived from the general and colorectal surgery literature with only limited research having been conducted in gynecologic surgery primarily addressing the lack of need for drainage following lymphadenectomy.[67,68] Bowel anastomoses can be divided into nonpelvic, pelvic, and pelvic below the peritoneal reflection in terms of the risk for anastomotic leak and the corresponding need for prophylactic drainage. With the exception of the bowel anastomoses below the peritoneal reflection where there may be a potential benefit in prophylactic drainage for a short period postoperatively,[69–72] data do not support the routine use of prophylactic drainage following bowel resection[70,73–76]; of note, only one study was specific to gynecologic oncology and did not support the routine use of drains following bowel resection in patients with ovarian cancer.[65] Peritoneal drains should be considered within an ERAS protocol when there is increased likelihood for pelvic collections postoperatively, bleeding concerns despite meticulous hemostasis, or very low anterior resections with no concurrent temporary bowel diversion.[77]

Postoperative

Early postoperative feeding

Early feeding is considered resumption of oral fluid and solid intake within 24 hours after surgery. Within the ERAS pathway, the patient is typically allowed to drink fluids upon recovering from anesthesia and encouraged to resume regular diet upon arrival at the floor. Central to the ERAS concept, oral intake is merely encouraged, neither forced nor withheld; the patient dictates the amount and type of oral intake. Several randomized trials in gynecologic surgery provide evidence in favor of early postoperative feeding.[63,78–81] These studies indicate that early feeding results in earlier return of bowel function and shorter LOS with no change in postoperative complications, including pulmonary complications, anastomotic leak, and wound healing.[82,83] It is important to note that, although few studies have linked early feeding to a small increase in postoperative nausea, this association did not extend to vomiting, abdominal distention, or need for NGT use.[80,81,83] Importantly, patients continued to rate their satisfaction with early feeding protocols very highly.[84]

Early mobilization

Early mobilization is a key component in ERAS protocols. It has been stipulated that it protects against muscle loss and deconditioning by avoiding prolonged bed rest and immobility, helps reduce pulmonary and venous thromboembolic complications, improves insulin resistance, and contributes to shortening hospitalizations.[85,86] Research has shown that daily use of a diary with postoperative day-specific mobilization goals along with active engagement of patients and nursing staff in registering, whether these goals were being achieved or not, increased the rate of successful implementation of early mobilization protocols and was associated with a trend toward shorter hospitalization.[85,87]

Early urinary catheter removal

ERAS protocols call for removal of urinary catheters within 24 hours following surgery, with some advocating for even earlier removal. In a recent randomized prospective study on timing of urinary catheter removal following gynecologic surgery, Ind and colleagues[88] compared midnight removal (removal of urinary catheter at midnight on the day of surgery) to morning removal (removal of urinary catheter at 06:00 AM the day after surgery). They observed that patients, who had their catheter removed at midnight, required a shorter time to first void, were passing a larger volume of urine at first void, required less frequent recatheterization for urinary retention, and had a shorter hospital LOS. A meta-analysis including RCTs from a wide range of specialties reached similar conclusions.[89] An argument toward routine removal immediately after surgery in laparotomies does not appear to be substantiated based on a recent study comparing removal of urinary catheter immediately after surgery, 6 hours, or 24 hours postoperatively following uncomplicated total abdominal hysterectomy.[90] The intermediate removal group (removal of catheter 6 hours postoperatively) was superior to the immediate group (removal at the end of surgery) in terms of less frequent need for recatheterization and superior to the delayed group (removal within 24 hours postoperatively) in terms of less frequent urinary tract infections, earlier ambulation, and shorter hospital LOS.

Perioperative pain management

Excellent perioperative pain management is one of the most central components within the ERAS pathways. The goal is to maximize efficacy of pain control while minimizing the amount of opioids used. Opioid use has traditionally been associated with increased PONV, impairment of bowel function, delayed mobilization due to altered mental sensorium, and increased pulmonary morbidity due to depression of respiratory drive. ERAS protocols aim to achieve this goal with a combination of a multimodal pharmacologic pain regimen and regional analgesia.

Multimodal pharmacologic analgesia The efficacy of this approach is based on the ability of 2 or more medication to act synergistically.[91] Use of nonsteroidal anti-inflammatory drugs (NSAIDs/COX-2 inhibitors) has been proven effective in controlling postoperative pain while reducing opioid requirements, reducing PONV, and increasing patient satisfaction[35,92,93]; furthermore, a combination of NSAIDs with paracetamol offers superior analgesia compared with either drug alone.[34] The use of NSAIDs in the immediate postoperative period was initially received with reservation because of preliminary data suggesting that their use may be associated with increased risk of postoperative complications including anastomotic leak.[94–97] However, in a large, multicenter study across 109 centers in the United Kingdom, the investigators failed to detect any association between early use of NSAIDs and anastomotic leak; in fact, treatment with NSAIDs was associated with a statistically significant 28% reduction in overall complications.[98] Furthermore, despite initial concerns over increased risk of postoperative bleeding following ketorolac use, Gobble and colleagues[99] conducted a meta-analysis of 27 RCTs incorporating 2314 patients and concluded that postoperative bleeding was not statistically increased with ketorolac and that ketorolac offered pain control that was superior to controls and equivalent to opioids.

Regional analgesia Regional analgesic techniques are important adjuncts to the multi-modal pharmacologic analgesic regimen within the ERAS pathways in order to achieve adequate pain control while decreasing opioid requirements and, ultimately, hastening recovery. These techniques include thoracic epidural analgesia (TEA), transversus abdominis plane (TAP) blocks, wound infiltration with local anesthetic, and intraperitoneal local anesthetic (IPLA).

Thoracic epidural analgesia TEA is considered standard of care in the vast majority of ERAS pathways from the colorectal, thoracic, vascular, hepatobiliary, and urologic literature.[100,101] TEA has consistently been found to be superior to IV opioid PCA and has been associated with decreased PONV, earlier return of bowel function, and decreased postoperative insulin resistance. In contrast, data on the efficacy of TEA in gynecologic surgery are conflicting. Although de Leon-Casasola and colleagues[102] concluded that TEA after radical hysterectomy resulted in a decrease in the duration of postoperative ileus leading to earlier hospital discharge, other investigators failed to prove benefit in terms of shortened length of hospitalization despite superior pain control,[103] and others failed to prove there was any benefit in pain management.[104] Important additional considerations when contemplating use of TEA in gynecologic surgery are the difficulty with proper management of TEAs and the high reported failure rate up to 30%.[105] For example, hypotension secondary to sympathetic blockade following TEA commonly ensues and, if it is inappropriately treated with fluid boluses instead of vasopressors, fluid overload can undermine the benefits of the fluid restrictive approach. Moreover, TEA can sometimes hinder early mobilization and early urinary catheter removal. Under such circumstances, TEA may result in impaired recovery and paradoxic prolongation of hospital LOS.

In the authors' experience, strict adherence to a multimodal pharmacologic regimen postoperatively (scheduled paracetamol and ketorolac/NSAIDs along with opioids on an as-needed basis), combined with wound infiltration with local anesthetic before incision closure, resulted in stable to improved pain scores, 80% reduction in the use of opioids in the first 48 hours, a 7-fold decrease in IV PCA use, and a 4-day reduction in hospital LOS despite omitting use of TEA.[84]

Transversus abdominis plane block TAP block is an analgesic technique that involves infiltration of local anesthetic in the plane between the internal oblique and transversus abdominis muscles, first described by Rafi in 2001.[106] Among several modifications described since its first use, 2 important advancements consist of performing TAP blocks under ultrasound guidance to improve accuracy of delivery of local anesthetic at the right plane[107] as well as the open surgically placed approach, whereby delivery of local anesthetic at the right plane is performed through direct visualization intraoperatively at the time of abdominal wound closure.[108,109] TAP blocks have been used in patients undergoing a wide range of abdominal surgeries including large bowel resection via a midline abdominal incision, caesarean delivery via the Pfannenstiel incision, abdominal hysterectomy via a transverse lower abdominal wall incision, open appendectomy, and laparoscopic cholecystectomy. They have been proven safe and appear to reduce postoperative opioid requirements and PONV and improve postoperative pain management.[110] A meta-analysis of 6 RCTs comparing TAP blocks to no block or placebo block in patients undergoing open gynecologic surgery found that their use was associated with superior pain management and decreased opioid requirements up to 24 hours postoperatively.[111] Nonetheless, the investigators concluded that data remain limited and that future studies should be undertaken before conclusive recommendations can be safely made. Per current guidelines for postoperative care following open general gynecologic surgery from the ERAS Society, TAP blocks may be considered in patients who have undergone general anesthesia without neuraxial blockade.[112]

Wound infiltration Wound infiltration of surgical site with local anesthetic is recognized as a safe, easy-to-perform, and effective method of postoperative pain management.[113] Given its limited duration of action of an average of 8 hours, delivery systems such as elastometric pumps have been used for continuous wound infiltration (CIW) with local anesthetic. In a meta-analysis of 44 RCTs, Liu and colleagues[114] found that CIW resulted in reduced pain scores and opioid use across most of the surgical specialties. Although clinical outcomes such as opioid-related side effects, patient satisfaction, and LOS were infrequently assessed for each surgical group, CIW was associated with decreased PONV and shorter LOS when analyzing all data together. In contrast, data from the gynecologic literature are conflicting with few groups showing clinical benefit in terms of pain control and opioid use,[115,116] while others failing to demonstrate any benefit.[117–119] Importantly, these systems are often difficult to use, and catheters can be easily dislodged and can lead to surgical site infections. An alternative method to achieve longer duration of postoperative pain control consists of wound infiltration with a long-acting anesthetic medication, called liposomal bupivacaine. This medication uses a delivery platform that releases the drug slowly over 72 to 96 hours.[120] An increasing number of studies indicate that a single-dose surgical site infiltration with liposomal bupivacaine at the end of the procedure provides effective local analgesia up to 72 hours and results in a significant reduction in opioid use following hemorrhoidectomy, bunionectomy, breast augmentation, inguinal hernia repair, and total knee arthroplasty.[121–124] The authors' group recently conducted a study on its efficacy against regular bupivacaine within an established ERAS protocol in gynecologic surgery and found that its use resulted in a significant decrease in PCA use as well as opioid requirements while maintaining adequate pain control (Kalogera E, Bakkum-Gamez JN, Dowdy SC. Liposomal Bupivacaine Reduces Total and IV Opioid Requirements after Laparotomy for Gynecologic Malignancies. Submitted for publication).

Intraperitoneal local anesthetic IPLA involves instilling local anesthetic solution into the peritoneal cavity in order to block visceral vagal afferent signaling that gives rise to both painful and nonpainful sensations in order to further reduce postoperative pain. There are only limited data on the use of IPLA following abdominal hysterectomy, indicating that it may reduce opioid requirements and possibly reduce postoperative pain, but its effect appears to be limited to the immediate postoperative period up to 4 hours after surgery.[125,126]

Considerations specific to vaginal hysterectomy Per current guidelines from the ERAS Society, in addition to multimodal pharmacologic analgesia, local anesthetic infiltration in the form of paracervical block or intrathecal morphine may be considered following vaginal hysterectomy. Limited data indicate that these approaches may be associated with a small effect in reducing pain and opioid requirements and may facilitate early mobilization.[112]

Considerations specific to minimally invasive gynecologic surgery Per current guidelines from the ERAS Society, multimodal pharmacologic analgesia should be used following minimally invasive gynecologic surgery. However, there is not enough evidence to support the routine use of TAP blocks or IPLA in this setting. TEA may prolong hospitalization without improving outcomes.[112]

Postoperative fluid management

Similar to preoperative and intraoperative fluid goals, euvolemia should be maintained in the postoperative period. Patients are allowed to drink immediately after surgery, and IV fluids are discontinued once they have demonstrated ability to maintain oral hydration, typically once they have had at least 500 mL of oral fluid intake. In the ERAS pathways, it is very rare that IV fluids will be required beyond 12 to 24 hours postoperatively. Even in the immediate postoperative period, the rate of IV fluid administration is kept at a minimum, no higher than 1.2 mL/kg, oftentimes much lower.[127] Toward preventing fluid overload, fluid boluses should be used cautiously and always taking into consideration the overall clinical picture. It is important to recognize that urine output as low as 20 mL/h is a normal response to surgical stress and does not require intervention.[128,129] Balanced crystalloids (ie, Ringer lactate), which are solutions with an electrolyte concentration similar to plasma, are preferred to 0.9% normal saline in order to prevent hyperchloremic acidosis.[130]

Laxative use and prevention of postoperative ileus

ERAS protocols incorporate early use of laxatives with the goal to hasten return of gastrointestinal function. One of the first studies in gynecologic oncology on aggressive postoperative bowel stimulation studied the use of milk of magnesia on postoperative day 1 combined with biscolic suppositories on postoperative day 2 following radical hysterectomy.[131] This regimen resulted in a 4-day decrease in LOS with no associated untoward effects. The investigators reached similar conclusions when they completed a follow-up study during which they studied the combination of early feeding followed by Fleet Phospho-soda on postoperative day 1 in patients undergoing radical hysterectomy for cervical cancer.[132] Hansen and colleagues[133] observed that oral bowel stimulation with osmotic laxatives within 6 hours after abdominal hysterectomy resulted in earlier time to first bowel movement compared with placebo (45 hours vs 69 hours; $P<.001$) with no change in pain scores, PONV, antiemetic, or opioid use.

Several additional interventions have been investigated toward preventing postoperative ileus. Chewing gum early in the postoperative period following total abdominal hysterectomy with pelvic and para-aortic lymphadenectomy is inexpensive, well-tolerated, and proven to hasten return of bowel function.[134] Herzog and colleagues[135] performed a randomized trial of Alvimopan, a novel peripherally acting mu-opioid receptor antagonist. It was found to be safe and well-tolerated and improved gastrointestinal recovery by reducing time to first bowel movement by 22 hours as well as increasing frequency and improving quality of bowel movement in patients undergoing simple total abdominal hysterectomy. In contrast to Alvimopan, there is little to no evidence to support the use of other prokinetics in this setting.[136]

HASTENING POSTOPERATIVE RECOVERY

An increasing number of investigators from the United States, Europe, and Australia have published their experience with ERAS programs in a wide range of settings, including tertiary and nontertiary hospitals. ERAS protocols have been universally successful in decreasing length of hospital stay without an increase in complication and readmission rates.

Enhanced Recovery After Surgery and Benign Abdominal Hysterectomy

Miller and colleagues[137] compared 123 patients undergoing open gynecologic surgery for nonmalignant disease via abdominal incision under an ERAS protocol to 100 patients who had undergone similar procedures before ERAS adoption. Median

LOS was statistically significantly shorter by 1 day in the ERAS cohort with a median LOS of 2 days (interquartile range 1.0–3.0) versus 3 days (2.5–3.0) in the pre-ERAS cohort ($P<.001$). About a third of patients treated under the ERAS pathway were discharged on postoperative day 1, representing a 4-fold increase in early discharges compared with prior practice (ERAS vs pre-ERAS 34% vs 7%, respectively; $P<.001$). The rate of 30-day readmissions was unchanged between the 2 practices (ERAS vs pre-ERAS 10% vs 13%, respectively; $P = .49$). Interestingly, inhaled general anesthesia was the only independent factor associated with decreased odds for early discharge.

Wijk and colleagues[138] evaluated 85 patients undergoing abdominal hysterectomy for benign or malignant indications under ERAS against 120 patients undergoing the same type of surgery before ERAS. Of note, only unilateral or bilateral salpingo-oophorectomy and omentectomy could be performed in addition to hysterectomy; patients with additional pelvic surgery were not included in this study. A higher proportion of patients were discharged within 2 days after ERAS establishment (ERAS vs pre-ERAS 73% vs 56%, respectively; $P = .012$). LOS was decreased from a mean of 2.6 days to 2.3 days ($P = .011$). Reoperation, complication, and 30-day readmission rates did not differ between the 2 practices.

Investigators evaluating all types of hysterectomies (open, laparoscopic, vaginal) as one group reached similar conclusions. Narang and colleagues[139] observed that patients undergoing hysterectomy or myomectomy (open or laparoscopic) following ERAS implementation had a mean LOS of 3.6 days compared with 5.1 days in the pre-ERAS cohort, a 29% reduction. Readmission rates were unchanged. Torbe and Louden[140] and Sjetne and colleagues[141] compared patients undergoing hysterectomy (open, laparoscopic, vaginal) before and after integration of an ERAS pathway and observed a 1-day reduction in mean LOS (2.7 vs 1.8 days, and 4.7 vs 3.4 days, respectively).

Descriptive studies of cohorts of patients undergoing benign abdominal hysterectomy under ERAS protocols reported similar reductions in LOS. Carter and colleagues[142,143] reported a medial LOS of 3 days with 42% of patients being discharged by postoperative day 2. Similarly, Moller and colleagues[144] observed median LOS of 2 days and Chowdhury and colleagues[145] observed median LOS of 2.64 days. Complications and readmission rates in these studies were comparable with rates reported by prior investigators.

Enhanced Recovery After Surgery and Vaginal Hysterectomy

Yoong and colleagues[146] compared 50 patients who underwent vaginal hysterectomy (18% with concomitant repairs) after implementation of ERAS to 50 patients who underwent the same procedure (20% with concomitant repairs) before ERAS. They noted a 51.6% reduction in median LOS (22.0 vs 45.5 hours; $P<.01$) without adversely affecting the readmission rate or the number of emergency department (ED) visits after dismissal. There was a 5-fold increase in the number of patients being discharged within 24 hours under the ERAS protocol compared with the pre-ERAS practice (78% vs 15.6%; $P<.05$). Other descriptive studies on simple vaginal hysterectomy without other concomitant surgery corroborate these findings with mean or median LOS ranging from 1.0 to 1.8 days[144,145,147] with stable complication and readmission rates.

In the authors' study of ERAS,[84] they studied patients undergoing pelvic organ prolapse surgery, which included vaginal hysterectomy with concomitant repairs or posthysterectomy pelvic floor repair; isolated vaginal hysterectomies were excluded. Despite more extensive vaginal surgery compared with the Yoong and colleagues study, similar conclusions were reached. Almost half of the ERAS cohort (46.1%) were discharged on postoperative day 1 compared with only 6.5% of women in the pre-ERAS cohort (*P*<.01) with no change in the 30-day readmission and postoperative complication rate. Other investigators who studied implementation of ERAS pathways in the same type of procedures reported rates of discharge on postoperative day 1 as high as 93.1%.[148–150]

Enhanced Recovery After Surgery and Laparoscopic Hysterectomy

Although the feasibility and safety of same-day discharge following laparoscopic hysterectomy has been studied before the introduction of the ERAS pathways in gynecologic surgery,[151–153] ERAS pathways can hasten convalescence, shorten hospital LOS, and contribute toward safely achieving the goal of same-day discharge.

Minig and colleagues[154] evaluated the clinical outcomes of 88 patients undergoing laparoscopic hysterectomy for both benign and malignant indications under an ERAS pathway in Spain where the predominant culture is for the patients to remain in the hospital for at least 2 to 3 days, even after minimally invasive surgery. Although almost 80% of patients were fit for same-day discharge, only 27% were discharged the day of surgery due to patient preference; this highlights the importance of preoperative patient education and counseling. Eighty-five percent of patients were discharged by postoperative day 1. Readmission rate was stable compared with published literature, and the ED visits (13%) occurred at least 4 days after discharge and were not related to the ERAS protocol. Johnston and colleagues[155] noted similar results among patients undergoing laparoscopic hysterectomy for both benign and malignant indications: 74% of patients were discharged on postoperative day 1 (49% within 24 hours). These results are consistent with other published studies reporting median LOS between 1 to 2 days following laparoscopic hysterectomy under ERAS pathways.[145,148,156,157]

HEALTH ECONOMICS

In the current era of rapidly expanding health care costs, the value of new interventions should be critically examined. It has previously been suggested from the colorectal literature that implementation of ERAS protocols is associated with significant cost reductions,[158] primarily as a function of the resultant decrease in LOS. Only a few investigators have studied cost changes following implementation of ERAS protocols in benign gynecologic surgery. Furthermore, these reports focus almost exclusively on benign vaginal surgery.

The only 2 studies studying costs that include patients who underwent abdominal hysterectomy are from Narang and colleagues[139] (open or laparoscopic hysterectomy or myomectomy) and Torbe and Louden[140] (vaginal, laparoscopic, or abdominal hysterectomy). In the first study, the investigators reported a cost saving of $495 per stay per patient based on the reduction of LOS following ERAS adoption. In the latter study, there were 27 bed days saved among 31 patients being treated under the ERAS protocol over only 2 months, equating to a saving of $285 per patient.

Introduction of ERAS in pelvic organ prolapse surgery (posthysterectomy pelvic floor repair or vaginal hysterectomy with repairs) in the authors' practice resulted in $697.29 cost-saving per patient.[84] Similar but less impressive cost reduction was noted by Yoong and colleagues[146] after ERAS in patients undergoing vaginal hysterectomy (only approximately 20% with concurrent vaginal repair surgery). In their protocol, there were added expenses associated with formalized patient education in the form of a 1-hour gynecology class that used an ERAS-specialized nurse; these costs were ultimately offset by the reduction in the LOS, still resulting in a cost saving of $153 per patient.

HEALTH-RELATED QUALITY OF LIFE AND PATIENT SATISFACTION

The importance of preserving patient's quality of life while trying to achieve superior clinical outcomes has been increasingly recognized in clinical and surgical practice. Quality of life is particularly relevant for gynecologic patients because they are faced with sensitive issues, such as altered sexual function, loss of fertility, and disruption of normal anatomy of the female reproductive track.[159–161] ERAS pathways have been associated with improvement in patient-reported outcomes, improved quality of life, and excellent patient satisfaction.

De Groot and colleagues[162] considered successful functional recovery to have been achieved when the patient was able to tolerate general diet, mobilize independently, and have good control of postoperative pain with oral analgesia. They noted that the ERAS protocol resulted in earlier independent mobilization by 3 days, earlier oral fluid intake and ability to tolerate general diet by 2 days, as well as ability to have good control of postoperative pain with oral medication by 1 day. On the basis of these criteria, return to functional recovery was achieved 3 days earlier with the ERAS pathway compared with traditional perioperative care (3 days vs 6 days; $P<.001$). Meyer and colleagues[163] did not observe any change in the most highly rated patient-reported symptoms, which include fatigue, abdominal pain, and overall surgical pain. Specifically, pain scores were no different between pre-ERAS and post-ERAS patients despite a significant reduction in the amount of opioid medication required to treat postoperative pain. In contrast, they observed improvement in the severity of nausea, sleep disturbance, constipation, urinary urgency, and difficulty with memory during hospitalization. These findings are consistent with previously published studies on ERAS pathway in gynecologic surgery.[84,149]

Patient satisfaction following ERAS-associated perioperative care has consistently been reported as high. In one study by Ottesen and colleagues,[149] 92.7% of the patients stated that their hospitalization was "as expected," "easier than expected," or "much easier than expected." Most patients were satisfied with their hospital LOS; only a small percentage of patients of less than 5% (2/41) reported feeling "a little pressure put on them toward discharge," among which one was discharged on postoperative day 8. In a 0 to 10 scale of "how acceptable the program and advice had been," the median score was 10. Patient satisfaction rates have universally been reported high ranging from 75% to 95% across studies.[84,140,147,150,156]

SUMMARY

High-quality data support the safety and efficacy of ERAS pathways in enhancing postoperative recovery of patients undergoing gynecologic surgery. ERAS pathways have been consistently associated with improved postoperative outcomes including earlier return of gastrointestinal function, adequate pain management with reduced opioid use, shorter length of hospital stay, excellent patient satisfaction, and substantial cost reductions with no increase in complication or readmission rates. Successful implementation of an ERAS pathway requires a multidisciplinary and collaborative approach between surgeons, anesthesiologists, pharmacists, nursing staff, and physicians in training as well as active engagement of patients in the enhancement of their recovery. Systematic efforts are needed for active diffusion of the ERAS perioperative care model and should be considered standard of care in gynecologic surgery.

REFERENCES

1. Kehlet H. Multimodal approach to control postoperative pathophysiology and rehabilitation. Br J Anaesth 1997;78:606–17.
2. Kehlet H, Wilmore DW. Evidence-based surgical care and the evolution of fast-track surgery. Ann Surg 2008;248:189–98.
3. Kehlet H. Labat lecture 2005: surgical stress and postoperative outcome-from here to where? Reg Anesth Pain Med 2006;31:47–52.
4. Wilmore DW. From Cuthbertson to fast-track surgery: 70 years of progress in reducing stress in surgical patients. Ann Surg 2002;236:643–8.
5. Adamina M, Kehlet H, Tomlinson GA, et al. Enhanced recovery pathways optimize health outcomes and resource utilization: a meta-analysis of randomized controlled trials in colorectal surgery. Surgery 2011;149:830–40.
6. Anderson AD, McNaught CE, MacFie J, et al. Randomized clinical trial of multimodal optimization and standard perioperative surgical care. Br J Surg 2003; 90:1497–504.
7. Khan S, Wilson T, Ahmed J, et al. Quality of life and patient satisfaction with enhanced recovery protocols. Colorectal Dis 2010;12:1175–82.
8. Khoo CK, Vickery CJ, Forsyth N, et al. A prospective randomized controlled trial of multimodal perioperative management protocol in patients undergoing elective colorectal resection for cancer. Ann Surg 2007;245:867–72.
9. Lovely JK, Maxson PM, Jacob AK, et al. Case-matched series of enhanced versus standard recovery pathway in minimally invasive colorectal surgery. Br J Surg 2012;99:120–6.
10. Sammour T, Zargar-Shoshtari K, Bhat A, et al. A programme of Enhanced Recovery After Surgery (ERAS) is a cost-effective intervention in elective colonic surgery. N Z Med J 2010;123:61–70.
11. Spanjersberg WR, Reurings J, Keus F, et al. Fast track surgery versus conventional recovery strategies for colorectal surgery. Cochrane Database Syst Rev 2011;(2):CD007635.
12. Department of Health. Enhanced recovery partnership programme, report March 2011. Available at: http://www.dh.gov.uk/prod_consum_dh/groups/dh_digitalassets/documents/digitalasset/dh_. Accessed February 25, 2016.
13. Knott A, Pathak S, McGrath JS, et al. Consensus views on implementation and measurement of enhanced recovery after surgery in England: Delphi study. BMJ Open 2012;2:1V.
14. Varadhan KK, Neal KR, Dejong CH, et al. The enhanced recovery after surgery (ERAS) pathway for patients undergoing major elective open colorectal surgery: a meta-analysis of randomized controlled trials. Clin Nutr 2010;29:434–40.
15. Halaszynski TM, Juda R, Silverman DG. Optimizing postoperative outcomes with efficient preoperative assessment and management. Crit Care Med 2004; 32:S76–86.
16. Callesen T, Klarskov B, Bech K, et al. Short convalescence after inguinal herniorrhaphy with standardised recommendations: duration and reasons for delayed return to work. Eur J Surg 1999;165:236–41.
17. Soop M, Nygren J, Myrenfors P, et al. Preoperative oral carbohydrate treatment attenuates immediate postoperative insulin resistance. Am J Physiol Endocrinol Metab 2001;280:E576–83.
18. Greisen J, Juhl CB, Grofte T, et al. Acute pain induces insulin resistance in humans. Anesthesiology 2001;95:578–84.

19. Svanfeldt M, Thorell A, Brismar K, et al. Effects of 3 days of "postoperative" low caloric feeding with or without bed rest on insulin sensitivity in healthy subjects. Clin Nutr 2003;22:31–8.
20. Brady M, Kinn S, Stuart P. Preoperative fasting for adults to prevent perioperative complications. Cochrane Database Syst Rev 2003;(4):CD004423.
21. American Society of Anesthesiologists Committee. Practice guidelines for preoperative fasting and the use of pharmacologic agents to reduce the risk of pulmonary aspiration: application to healthy patients undergoing elective procedures: an updated report by the American Society of Anesthesiologists Committee on Standards and Practice Parameters. Anesthesiology 2011;114: 495–511.
22. Yuill KA, Richardson RA, Davidson HI, et al. The administration of an oral carbohydrate-containing fluid prior to major elective upper-gastrointestinal surgery preserves skeletal muscle mass postoperatively–a randomised clinical trial. Clin Nutr 2005;24:32–7.
23. Mathur S, Plank LD, McCall JL, et al. Randomized controlled trial of preoperative oral carbohydrate treatment in major abdominal surgery. Br J Surg 2010;97: 485–94.
24. Nygren J, Thorell A, Ljungqvist O. Preoperative oral carbohydrate nutrition: an update. Curr Opin Clin Nutr Metab Care 2001;4:255–9.
25. Fanning J, Valea FA. Perioperative bowel management for gynecologic surgery. Am J Obstet Gynecol 2011;205:309–14.
26. Arnold A, Aitchison LP, Abbott J. Preoperative mechanical bowel preparation for abdominal, laparoscopic, and vaginal surgery: a systematic review. J Minim Invasive Gynecol 2015;22:737–52.
27. Siedhoff MT, Clark LH, Hobbs KA, et al. Mechanical bowel preparation before laparoscopic hysterectomy: a randomized controlled trial. Obstet Gynecol 2014;123:562–7.
28. Morris MS, Graham LA, Chu DI, et al. Oral antibiotic bowel preparation significantly reduces surgical site infection rates and readmission rates in elective colorectal surgery. Ann Surg 2015;261:1034–40.
29. Toneva GD, Deierhoi RJ, Morris M, et al. Oral antibiotic bowel preparation reduces length of stay and readmissions after colorectal surgery. J Am Coll Surg 2013;216:756–62 [discussion: 762–3].
30. Kantartzis KL, Shepherd JP. The use of mechanical bowel preparation in laparoscopic gynecologic surgery: a decision analysis. Am J Obstet Gynecol 2015;213:721.e1–5.
31. Turan A, Karamanlioglu B, Memis D, et al. The analgesic effects of gabapentin after total abdominal hysterectomy. Anesth Analg 2004;98:1370–3.
32. Fassoulaki A, Stamatakis E, Petropoulos G, et al. Gabapentin attenuates late but not acute pain after abdominal hysterectomy. Eur J Anaesthesiol 2006;23: 136–41.
33. Ajori L, Nazari L, Mazloomfard MM, et al. Effects of gabapentin on postoperative pain, nausea and vomiting after abdominal hysterectomy: a double blind randomized clinical trial. Arch Gynecol Obstet 2012;285:677–82.
34. Ong CK, Seymour RA, Lirk P, et al. Combining paracetamol (acetaminophen) with nonsteroidal antiinflammatory drugs: a qualitative systematic review of analgesic efficacy for acute postoperative pain. Anesth Analg 2010;110:1170–9.
35. Maund E, McDaid C, Rice S, et al. Paracetamol and selective and non-selective non-steroidal anti-inflammatory drugs for the reduction in morphine-related side-effects after major surgery: a systematic review. Br J Anaesth 2011;106:292–7.

36. Gupta A, Stierer T, Zuckerman R, et al. Comparison of recovery profile after ambulatory anesthesia with propofol, isoflurane, sevoflurane and desflurane: a systematic review. Anesth Analg 2004;98:632–41.

37. White PF, O'Hara JF, Roberson CR, et al. The impact of current antiemetic practices on patient outcomes: a prospective study on high-risk patients. Anesth Analg 2008;107:452–8.

38. Apfel CC, Korttila K, Abdalla M, et al. A factorial trial of six interventions for the prevention of postoperative nausea and vomiting. N Engl J Med 2004;350: 2441–51.

39. Apfel CC, Heidrich FM, Jukar-Rao S, et al. Evidence-based analysis of risk factors for postoperative nausea and vomiting. Br J Anaesth 2012;109:742–53.

40. Borendal Wodlin N, Nilsson L, Kjolhede P. The impact of mode of anaesthesia on postoperative recovery from fast-track abdominal hysterectomy: a randomised clinical trial. BJOG 2011;118:299–308.

41. Acheson N, Crawford R. The impact of mode of anaesthesia on postoperative recovery from fast-track abdominal hysterectomy: a randomised clinical trial. BJOG 2011;118:271–3.

42. Carli F, Kehlet H, Baldini G, et al. Evidence basis for regional anesthesia in multidisciplinary fast-track surgical care pathways. Reg Anesth Pain Med 2011;36: 63–72.

43. Kurz A, Sessler DI, Lenhardt R. Perioperative normothermia to reduce the incidence of surgical-wound infection and shorten hospitalization. Study of Wound Infection and Temperature Group. N Engl J Med 1996;334:1209–15.

44. Rajagopalan S, Mascha E, Na J, et al. The effects of mild perioperative hypothermia on blood loss and transfusion requirement. Anesthesiology 2008;108: 71–7.

45. Scott EM, Buckland R. A systematic review of intraoperative warming to prevent postoperative complications. AORN J 2006;83:1090–104, 1107–13.

46. Wong PF, Kumar S, Bohra A, et al. Randomized clinical trial of perioperative systemic warming in major elective abdominal surgery. Br J Surg 2007;94:421–6.

47. Galvao CM, Marck PB, Sawada NO, et al. A systematic review of the effectiveness of cutaneous warming systems to prevent hypothermia. J Clin Nurs 2009; 18:627–36.

48. Perez-Protto S, Sessler DI, Reynolds LF, et al. Circulating-water garment or the combination of a circulating-water mattress and forced-air cover to maintain core temperature during major upper-abdominal surgery. Br J Anaesth 2010; 105:466–70.

49. MacKay G, Fearon K, McConnachie A, et al. Randomized clinical trial of the effect of postoperative intravenous fluid restriction on recovery after elective colorectal surgery. Br J Surg 2006;93:1469–74.

50. Nisanevich V, Felsenstein I, Almogy G, et al. Effect of intraoperative fluid management on outcome after intraabdominal surgery. Anesthesiology 2005;103: 25–32.

51. Varadhan KK, Lobo DN. A meta-analysis of randomised controlled trials of intravenous fluid therapy in major elective open abdominal surgery: getting the balance right. Proc Nutr Soc 2010;69:488–98.

52. Brandstrup B, Tonnesen H, Beier-Holgersen R, et al. Effects of intravenous fluid restriction on postoperative complications: comparison of two perioperative fluid regimens: a randomized assessor-blinded multicenter trial. Ann Surg 2003;238: 641–8.

53. Rahbari NN, Zimmermann JB, Schmidt T, et al. Meta-analysis of standard, restrictive and supplemental fluid administration in colorectal surgery. Br J Surg 2009;96:331–41.
54. Lobo DN, Bostock KA, Neal KR, et al. Effect of salt and water balance on recovery of gastrointestinal function after elective colonic resection: a randomised controlled trial. Lancet 2002;359:1812–8.
55. Gomez-Izquierdo JC, Feldman LS, Carli F, et al. Meta-analysis of the effect of goal-directed therapy on bowel function after abdominal surgery. Br J Surg 2015;102:577–89.
56. Gan TJ, Diemunsch P, Habib AS, et al. Consensus guidelines for the management of postoperative nausea and vomiting. Anesth Analg 2014;118:85–113.
57. Karanicolas PJ, Smith SE, Kanbur B, et al. The impact of prophylactic dexamethasone on nausea and vomiting after laparoscopic cholecystectomy: a systematic review and meta-analysis. Ann Surg 2008;248:751–62.
58. Carlisle JB, Stevenson CA. Drugs for preventing postoperative nausea and vomiting. Cochrane Database Syst Rev 2006;(3):CD004125.
59. Charlton S, Cyna AM, Middleton P, et al. Perioperative transversus abdominis plane (TAP) blocks for analgesia after abdominal surgery. Cochrane Database Syst Rev 2010;(12):CD007705.
60. Antor MA, Uribe AA, Erminy-Falcon N, et al. The effect of transdermal scopolamine for the prevention of postoperative nausea and vomiting. Front Pharmacol 2014;5:55.
61. Nelson R, Edwards S, Tse B. Prophylactic nasogastric decompression after abdominal surgery. Cochrane Database Syst Rev 2007;(3):CD004929.
62. Cheatham ML, Chapman WC, Key SP, et al. A meta-analysis of selective versus routine nasogastric decompression after elective laparotomy. Ann Surg 1995; 221:469–76 [discussion: 476–8].
63. Cutillo G, Maneschi F, Franchi M, et al. Early feeding compared with nasogastric decompression after major oncologic gynecologic surgery: a randomized study. Obstet Gynecol 1999;93:41–5.
64. Nelson G, Altman AD, Nick A, et al. Guidelines for pre- and intra-operative care in gynecologic/oncology surgery: enhanced recovery after surgery (ERAS(R)) society recommendations - part I. Gynecol Oncol 2016;140:313–22.
65. Kalogera E, Dowdy SC, Mariani A, et al. Utility of closed suction pelvic drains at time of large bowel resection for ovarian cancer. Gynecol Oncol 2012;126: 391–6.
66. Karliczek A, Jesus EC, Matos D, et al. Drainage or nondrainage in elective colorectal anastomosis: a systematic review and meta-analysis. Colorectal Dis 2006; 8:259–65.
67. Charoenkwan K, Kietpeerakool C. Retroperitoneal drainage versus no drainage after pelvic lymphadenectomy for the prevention of lymphocyst formation in patients with gynaecological malignancies. Cochrane Database Syst Rev 2014;(6):CD007387.
68. Morice P, Lassau N, Pautier P, et al. Retroperitoneal drainage after complete Para-aortic lymphadenectomy for gynecologic cancer: a randomized trial. Obstet Gynecol 2001;97:243–7.
69. Hoffmann J, Shokouh-Amiri MH, Damm P, et al. A prospective, controlled study of prophylactic drainage after colonic anastomoses. Dis Colon Rectum 1987;30: 449–52.
70. Merad F, Yahchouchi E, Hay JM, et al. Prophylactic abdominal drainage after elective colonic resection and suprapromontory anastomosis: a multicenter

study controlled by randomization. French Associations for Surgical Research. Arch Surg 1998;133:309–14.

71. Tytherleigh MG, Bokey L, Chapuis PH, et al. Is a minor clinical anastomotic leak clinically significant after resection of colorectal cancer? J Am Coll Surg 2007; 205:648–53.

72. Vignali A, Fazio VW, Lavery IC, et al. Factors associated with the occurrence of leaks in stapled rectal anastomoses: a review of 1,014 patients. J Am Coll Surg 1997;185:105–13.

73. Hoffman MS, Zervose E. Colon resection for ovarian cancer: intraoperative decisions. Gynecol Oncol 2008;111:S56–65.

74. Jurado M, Alcazar JL, Baixauli J, et al. Low colorectal anastomosis after pelvic exenteration for gynecologic malignancies: risk factors analysis for leakage. Int J Gynecol Cancer 2011;21:397–402.

75. Sagar PM, Hartley MN, Macfie J, et al. Randomized trial of pelvic drainage after rectal resection. Dis Colon Rectum 1995;38:254–8.

76. Jesus EC, Karliczek A, Matos D, et al. Prophylactic anastomotic drainage for colorectal surgery. Cochrane Database Syst Rev 2004;(4):CD002100.

77. Lopes AD, Hall JR, Monaghan JM. Drainage following radical hysterectomy and pelvic lymphadenectomy: dogma or need? Obstet Gynecol 1995;86:960–3.

78. Minig L, Biffi R, Zanagnolo V, et al. Early oral versus "traditional" postoperative feeding in gynecologic oncology patients undergoing intestinal resection: a randomized controlled trial. Ann Surg Oncol 2009;16:1660–8.

79. Charoenkwan K, Phillipson G, Vutyavanich T. Early versus delayed (traditional) oral fluids and food for reducing complications after major abdominal gynaecologic surgery. Cochrane Database Syst Rev 2007;(4):CD004508.

80. Pearl ML, Valea FA, Fischer M, et al. A randomized controlled trial of early postoperative feeding in gynecologic oncology patients undergoing intra-abdominal surgery. Obstet Gynecol 1998;92:94–7.

81. Schilder JM, Hurteau JA, Look KY, et al. A prospective controlled trial of early postoperative oral intake following major abdominal gynecologic surgery. Gynecol Oncol 1997;67:235–40.

82. Han-Geurts IJ, Hop WC, Kok NF, et al. Randomized clinical trial of the impact of early enteral feeding on postoperative ileus and recovery. Br J Surg 2007;94: 555–61.

83. Lewis SJ, Egger M, Sylvester PA, et al. Early enteral feeding versus "nil by mouth" after gastrointestinal surgery: systematic review and meta-analysis of controlled trials. BMJ 2001;323:773–6.

84. Kalogera E, Bakkum-Gamez JN, Jankowski CJ, et al. Enhanced recovery in gynecologic surgery. Obstet Gynecol 2013;122:319–28.

85. van der Leeden M, Huijsmans R, Geleijn E, et al. Early enforced mobilisation following surgery for gastrointestinal cancer: feasibility and outcomes. Physiotherapy 2016;102:103–10.

86. Kehlet H, Wilmore DW. Multimodal strategies to improve surgical outcome. Am J Surg 2002;183:630–41.

87. Lassen K, Soop M, Nygren J, et al. Consensus review of optimal perioperative care in colorectal surgery: enhanced recovery after surgery (ERAS) group recommendations. Arch Surg 2009;144:961–9.

88. Ind TEJ, Brown R, Pyneeandee VM, et al. Midnight removal of urinary catheters—improved outcome after gynecological surgery. Int Urogynecol J 1993;4: 342–5.

89. Griffiths R, Fernandez R. Strategies for the removal of short-term indwelling urethral catheters in adults. Cochrane Database Syst Rev 2007;(2):CD004011.
90. Ahmed MR, Sayed Ahmed WA, Atwa KA, et al. Timing of urinary catheter removal after uncomplicated total abdominal hysterectomy: a prospective randomized trial. Eur J Obstet Gynecol Reprod Biol 2014;176:60–3.
91. Buvanendran A, Kroin JS. Multimodal analgesia for controlling acute postoperative pain. Curr Opin Anaesthesiol 2009;22:588–93.
92. Niruthisard S, Werawataganon T, Bunburaphong P, et al. Improving the analgesic efficacy of intrathecal morphine with parecoxib after total abdominal hysterectomy. Anesth Analg 2007;105:822–4.
93. Blackburn A, Stevens JD, Wheatley RG, et al. Balanced analgesia with intravenous ketorolac and patient-controlled morphine following lower abdominal surgery. J Clin Anesth 1995;7:103–8.
94. Bhangu A, Singh P, Fitzgerald JE, et al. Postoperative nonsteroidal anti-inflammatory drugs and risk of anastomotic leak: meta-analysis of clinical and experimental studies. World J Surg 2014;38:2247–57.
95. Klein M, Gogenur I, Rosenberg J. Postoperative use of non-steroidal anti-inflammatory drugs in patients with anastomotic leakage requiring reoperation after colorectal resection: cohort study based on prospective data. BMJ 2012;345: e6166.
96. Gorissen KJ, Benning D, Berghmans T, et al. Risk of anastomotic leakage with non-steroidal anti-inflammatory drugs in colorectal surgery. Br J Surg 2012;99: 721–7.
97. Holte K, Andersen J, Jakobsen DH, et al. Cyclo-oxygenase 2 inhibitors and the risk of anastomotic leakage after fast-track colonic surgery. Br J Surg 2009;96: 650–4.
98. STARSurg Collaborative. Impact of postoperative non-steroidal anti-inflammatory drugs on adverse events after gastrointestinal surgery. Br J Surg 2014; 101:1413–23.
99. Gobble RM, Hoang HL, Kachniarz B, et al. Ketorolac does not increase perioperative bleeding: a meta-analysis of randomized controlled trials. Plast Reconstr Surg 2014;133:741–55.
100. Gustafsson UO, Scott MJ, Schwenk W, et al. Guidelines for perioperative care in elective colonic surgery: Enhanced Recovery After Surgery (ERAS((R))) Society recommendations. World J Surg 2013;37:259–84.
101. Nygren J, Thacker J, Carli F, et al. Guidelines for perioperative care in elective rectal/pelvic surgery: Enhanced Recovery After Surgery (ERAS(R)) Society recommendations. Clin Nutr 2012;31:801–16.
102. de Leon-Casasola OA, Karabella D, Lema MJ. Bowel function recovery after radical hysterectomies: thoracic epidural bupivacaine-morphine versus intravenous patient-controlled analgesia with morphine: a pilot study. J Clin Anesth 1996;8:87–92.
103. Ferguson SE, Malhotra T, Seshan VE, et al. A prospective randomized trial comparing patient-controlled epidural analgesia to patient-controlled intravenous analgesia on postoperative pain control and recovery after major open gynecologic cancer surgery. Gynecol Oncol 2009;114:111–6.
104. Chen LM, Weinberg VK, Chen C, et al. Perioperative outcomes comparing patient controlled epidural versus intravenous analgesia in gynecologic oncology surgery. Gynecol Oncol 2009;115:357–61.
105. Ready LB. Acute pain: lessons learned from 25,000 patients. Reg Anesth Pain Med 1999;24:499–505.

106. Rafi AN. Abdominal field block: a new approach via the lumbar triangle. Anaesthesia 2001;56:1024–6.
107. Atim A, Bilgin F, Kilickaya O, et al. The efficacy of ultrasound-guided transversus abdominis plane block in patients undergoing hysterectomy. Anaesth Intensive Care 2011;39:630–4.
108. Bharti N, Kumar P, Bala I, et al. The efficacy of a novel approach to transversus abdominis plane block for postoperative analgesia after colorectal surgery. Anesth Analg 2011;112:1504–8.
109. Owen DJ, Harrod I, Ford J, et al. The surgical transversus abdominis plane block–a novel approach for performing an established technique. BJOG 2011;118:24–7.
110. Johns N, O'Neill S, Ventham NT, et al. Clinical effectiveness of transversus abdominis plane (TAP) block in abdominal surgery: a systematic review and meta-analysis. Colorectal Dis 2012;14:e635–42.
111. Champaneria R, Shah L, Geoghegan J, et al. Analgesic effectiveness of transversus abdominis plane blocks after hysterectomy: a meta-analysis. Eur J Obstet Gynecol Reprod Biol 2013;166:1–9.
112. Nelson G, Altman AD, Nick A, et al. Guidelines for postoperative care in gynecologic/oncology surgery: Enhanced Recovery After Surgery (ERAS) Society recommendations– part II. Gynecol Oncol 2016;140:323–32.
113. American Society of Anesthesiologists Task Force on Acute Pain Management. Practice guidelines for acute pain management in the perioperative setting: an updated report by the American Society of Anesthesiologists Task Force on Acute Pain Management. Anesthesiology 2012;116:248–73.
114. Liu SS, Richman JM, Thirlby RC, et al. Efficacy of continuous wound catheters delivering local anesthetic for postoperative analgesia: a quantitative and qualitative systematic review of randomized controlled trials. J Am Coll Surg 2006; 203:914–32.
115. Maric S, Banovic M, Sakic ZK, et al. Continuous wound infusion of levobupivacaine after total abdominal hysterectomy with bilateral salpingo-oophorectomy. Period Biol 2009;111:299–302.
116. Zohar E, Fredman B, Phillipov A, et al. The analgesic efficacy of patient-controlled bupivacaine wound instillation after total abdominal hysterectomy with bilateral salpingo-oophorectomy. Anesth Analg 2001;93:482–7, 4th contents page.
117. Kushner DM, LaGalbo R, Connor JP, et al. Use of a bupivacaine continuous wound infusion system in gynecologic oncology: a randomized trial. Obstet Gynecol 2005;106:227–33.
118. Leong WM, Lo WK, Chiu JW. Analgesic efficacy of continuous delivery of bupivacaine by an elastomeric balloon infusor after abdominal hysterectomy: a prospective randomised controlled trial. Aust N Z J Obstet Gynaecol 2002;42: 515–8.
119. Kristensen BB, Christensen DS, Ostergaard M, et al. Lack of postoperative pain relief after hysterectomy using preperitoneally administered bupivacaine. Reg Anesth Pain Med 1999;24:576–80.
120. Davidson EM, Barenholz Y, Cohen R, et al. High-dose bupivacaine remotely loaded into multivesicular liposomes demonstrates slow drug release without systemic toxic plasma concentrations after subcutaneous administration in humans. Anesth Analg 2010;110:1018–23.
121. Bramlett KW, Jones RK, Pink M, et al. A single administration of depobupivacaine intraoperatively provides analgesia and reduction in use of rescue opiates

compared with bupivacaine HCl in patients undergoing total knee arthroplasty [poster]. In: Presented at the XXXVI Biennial World Congress of the International College of Surgeons. Vienna, Austria; December 3–6, 2008.
122. Golf M, Daniels SE, Onel E. A phase 3, randomized, placebo-controlled trial of DepoFoam(R) bupivacaine (extended-release bupivacaine local analgesic) in bunionectomy. Adv Ther 2011;28:776–88.
123. Gorfine SR, Onel E, Patou G, et al. Bupivacaine extended-release liposome injection for prolonged postsurgical analgesia in patients undergoing hemorrhoidectomy: a multicenter, randomized, double-blind, placebo-controlled trial. Dis colon rectum 2011;54:1552–9.
124. Smoot JD, Bergese SD, Onel E, et al. The efficacy and safety of DepoFoam bupivacaine in patients undergoing bilateral, cosmetic, submuscular augmentation mammaplasty: a randomized, double-blind, active-control study. Aesthet Surg J 2012;32:69–76.
125. Perniola A, Gupta A, Crafoord K, et al. Intraabdominal local anaesthetics for postoperative pain relief following abdominal hysterectomy: a randomized, double-blind, dose-finding study. Eur J Anaesthesiol 2009;26:421–9.
126. Gupta A, Perniola A, Axelsson K, et al. Postoperative pain after abdominal hysterectomy: a double-blind comparison between placebo and local anesthetic infused intraperitoneally. Anesth Analg 2004;99:1173–9.
127. Royal College of Physicians. Intravenous fluid therapy: intravenous fluid therapy in adults in hospital. London: National Clinical Guideline Centre; 2013.
128. Dudley HF, Boling EA, Lequesne LP, et al. Studies on antidiuresis in surgery: effects of anesthesia, surgery and posterior pituitary antidiuretic hormone on water metabolism in man. Ann Surg 1954;140:354–67.
129. Srinivasa S, Hill AG. Perioperative fluid administration: historical highlights and implications for practice. Ann Surg 2012;256:1113–8.
130. Wilkes NJ, Woolf R, Mutch M, et al. The effects of balanced versus saline-based hetastarch and crystalloid solutions on acid-base and electrolyte status and gastric mucosal perfusion in elderly surgical patients. Anesth Analg 2001;93:811–6.
131. Fanning J, Yu-Brekke S. Prospective trial of aggressive postoperative bowel stimulation following radical hysterectomy. Gynecol Oncol 1999;73:412–4.
132. Kraus K, Fanning J. Prospective trial of early feeding and bowel stimulation after radical hysterectomy. Am J Obstet Gynecol 2000;182:996–8.
133. Hansen CT, Sorensen M, Moller C, et al. Effect of laxatives on gastrointestinal functional recovery in fast-track hysterectomy: a double-blind, placebo-controlled randomized study. Am J Obstet Gynecol 2007;196:311.e1–7.
134. Ertas IE, Gungorduk K, Ozdemir A, et al. Influence of gum chewing on postoperative bowel activity after complete staging surgery for gynecological malignancies: a randomized controlled trial. Gynecol Oncol 2013;131:118–22.
135. Herzog TJ, Coleman RL, Guerrieri JP Jr, et al. A double-blind, randomized, placebo-controlled phase III study of the safety of alvimopan in patients who undergo simple total abdominal hysterectomy. Am J Obstet Gynecol 2006;195:445–53.
136. Traut U, Brugger L, Kunz R, et al. Systemic prokinetic pharmacologic treatment for postoperative adynamic ileus following abdominal surgery in adults. Cochrane Database Syst Rev 2008;(1):CD004930.
137. Miller EC, McIsaac DI, Chaput A, et al. Increased postoperative day one discharges after implementation of a hysterectomy enhanced recovery pathway: a retrospective cohort study. Can J Anaesth 2015;62:451–60.

138. Wijk L, Franzen K, Ljungqvist O, et al. Implementing a structured Enhanced Recovery After Surgery (ERAS) protocol reduces length of stay after abdominal hysterectomy. Acta Obstet Gynecol Scand 2014;93:749–56.

139. Narang L, Mitchelmore S, Byrne H. Cost reduction and enhanced patient experience following the introduction of enhanced recovery programme in gynaecological surgery. BJOG 2013;120:439.

140. Torbe E, Louden K. An enhanced recovery programme for women undergoing hysterectomy. Int J Gynecol Obstet 2012;119:S690.

141. Sjetne IS, Krogstad U, Odegard S, et al. Improving quality by introducing enhanced recovery after surgery in a gynaecological department: consequences for ward nursing practice. Qual Saf Health Care 2009;18:236–40.

142. Carter J. Fast-track surgery in gynaecology and gynaecologic oncology: a review of a rolling clinical audit. ISRN Surg 2012;2012:368014.

143. Carter J, Szabo R, Sim WW, et al. Fast track surgery: a clinical audit. Aust N Z J Obstet Gynaecol 2010;50:159–63.

144. Moller C, Kehlet H, Friland SG, et al. Fast track hysterectomy. Eur J Obstet Gynecol Reprod Biol 2001;98:18–22.

145. Chowdhury P, Kadry M, Raslan F. Audit of the enhanced recovery programme for hysterectomy at West Middlesex University Hospital. BJOG 2012;119:230.

146. Yoong W, Sivashanmugarajan V, Relph S, et al. Can enhanced recovery pathways improve outcomes of vaginal hysterectomy? Cohort control study. J Minim Invasive Gynecol 2014;21:83–9.

147. Ulrich D, Bjelic-Radisic V, Bader A, et al. Fast-track hysterectomy: a pilot study. Arch Gynecol Obstet 2010;282:S122–3.

148. Smith Walker T, Hindley J, Stocker M. Introducing enhanced recovery into gynaecological surgery at a district general hospital. Gynecol Surg 2011;8:S204.

149. Ottesen M, Sorensen M, Rasmussen Y, et al. Fast track vaginal surgery. Acta Obstet Gynecol Scand 2002;81:138–46.

150. Mistrangelo E, Deltetto F, Febo G. Fast track surgery in urogynecology. Neurourol Urodyn 2011;30:7–8.

151. Perron-Burdick M, Yamamoto M, Zaritsky E. Same-day discharge after laparoscopic hysterectomy. Obstet Gynecol 2011;117:1136–41.

152. Schiavone MB, Herzog TJ, Ananth CV, et al. Feasibility and economic impact of same-day discharge for women who undergo laparoscopic hysterectomy. Am J Obstet Gynecol 2012;207:382.e1–9.

153. Lassen PD, Moeller-Larsen H, P DEN. Same-day discharge after laparoscopic hysterectomy. Acta Obstet Gynecol Scand 2012;91:1339–41.

154. Minig L, Chuang L, Patrono MG, et al. Clinical outcomes after fast-track care in women undergoing laparoscopic hysterectomy. Int J Gynaecol Obstet 2015;131:301–4.

155. Johnston C, Crawford N, Ahmed I, et al. Laparoscopic hysterectomy: evaluating and improving service through the enhanced recovery pathway. Gynecol Surg 2015;12(Suppl 1):S200.

156. Ali O, Moukarram H. Pathway of enhanced recovery for total laparoscopic hysterectomy, pilot study of 50 cases. J Minim Invasive Gynecol 2015;22(6):S216.

157. Kent A, Waters N, Mitchell W. Laparoscopic hysterectomy (LH) and enhanced recovery pathway (ERP). Gynecol Surg 2012;(Suppl 1):S10.

158. Lemanu DP, Singh PP, Stowers MD, et al. A systematic review to assess cost effectiveness of enhanced recovery after surgery programmes in colorectal surgery. Colorectal Dis 2014;16:338–46.

159. Anderson B, Lutgendorf S. Quality of life in gynecologic cancer survivors. CA Cancer J Clin 1997;47:218–25.
160. Cull A, Cowie VJ, Farquharson DI, et al. Early stage cervical cancer: psychosocial and sexual outcomes of treatment. Br J Cancer 1993;68:1216–20.
161. Auchincloss SS. After treatment. Psychosocial issues in gynecologic cancer survivorship. Cancer 1995;76:2117–24.
162. de Groot JJA, van Es LEJM, Maessen JMC, et al. Diffusion of enhanced recovery principles in gynecologic oncology surgery: is active implementation still necessary? Gynecol Oncol 2014;134:570–5.
163. Meyer L, Nick A, Shi Q, et al. Comparison of patient reported symptom burden pre- and postimplementation of an enhanced recovery pathway (ERP) for gynecologic surgery. Int J Gynecol Cancer 2015;25(Suppl 2):40.

Surgical Simulation and Competency

Shunaha Kim-Fine, MD, MS*, Erin A. Brennand, MD

KEYWORDS

- Surgical training • Simulation • Competency • Hysterectomy • Education

KEY POINTS

- Simulation in surgical training is prevalent in obstetrics and gynecology training programs but not yet as part of a standardized curriculum.
- Evidence shows that simulation-based training improves knowledge and skill acquisition.
- Simulation-based competency assessment should specifically target the type of skills or knowledge to be assessed.
- When hysterectomy is viewed within a framework of increasing levels of competencies, different types of simulation can be used to help learners gain competencies until procedural mastery is achieved.

INTRODUCTION

In the 1800s, Dr Halsted at Johns Hopkins School of Medicine pioneered the first surgical training program in the United States. Surgeons were trained in the classical apprenticeship model of surgical training, and subsequent generations of surgeons were successfully trained in this model. However, since the 1990s, there have been several social and technological changes that questioned the philosophy of "see one, do one, teach one." These factors include concerns for patient safety, new duty hour restrictions for trainees, the introduction of new procedures and technologies, and the need for cost containment in the health care system.[1–4] All these factors culminate in an environment that may reduce teaching and learning opportunities in the operating room (OR) for trainees. Dimitris and colleagues[5] found that there has been a decrease in procedures performed and clinical encounters by surgical residents in the period after implementation of duty hour restrictions in the United States. At the same time, there has been a shift away from a time-based system of residency programs to a competency-based system. Specific to obstetrics and gynecology (OBGYN), resident hours are split between obstetric experience and gynecologic

Disclosures: No conflicts of interest.
Department of Obstetrics and Gynecology, University of Calgary, 29 Street NW, Calgary, Alberta T2N 2T9, Canada
* Corresponding author. Department of Obstetrics and Gynecology, Foothills Medical Centre, 4th Floor North Tower, 1403 29th Street Northwest, Calgary, Alberta T2N 2T9, Canada.
E-mail address: skima29@gmail.com

Obstet Gynecol Clin N Am 43 (2016) 575–590
http://dx.doi.org/10.1016/j.ogc.2016.04.007
0889-8545/16/$ – see front matter Crown Copyright © 2016 Published by Elsevier Inc. All rights reserved.

obgyn.theclinics.com

surgical training. Because so many hours are spent focusing on the acquisition of obstetric skills, residents in our specialty spend fewer months on surgical rotations per year than their counterparts in training programs of other surgical disciplines.[6]

Simulation has been proposed as a solution to the apparent conflict of improving patient safety while ensuring adequate opportunities for trainees to gain proficiency in surgical procedures. It has been shown that patients are more willing to allow trainees to perform procedures if they already have competency with simulators.[7] The ethics of allowing trainees to perform procedures is a complex balance of the principles of beneficence, nonmaleficence, and truth (**Fig. 1**). Although there is the need to provide best possible care, the patient more often believes such care is provided by the individual surgeon exclusively in the OR. In reality, such care is often provided in teaching centers by a combination of faculty and the surgical trainees, albeit under direct supervision of the surgeon. Surgical simulation can help ease the conflict between providing safe care, meeting the learning goals of trainees, and preserving truthfulness in the therapeutic relationship.

OPTIONS FOR SURGICAL SIMULATION

Simulation in surgery can take many forms (**Box 1**), which are described further below.

Animal and Human Cadaver Simulation

Animal and cadaver laboratories are the first examples of simulation in surgery. Advantages include high face validity in terms of anatomy, haptics, and tissue quality. However, changing values, ethics, and regulations around the use of animal and cadaveric tissue has resulted in much more expense and difficult access for such simulation. Many residency training programs may only be able to offer trainees exposure to either live animal or cadaver simulation laboratories and only infrequently during the course of their residency (Ari Sanders, MD, personal communication, 2016, Calgary, Alberta).

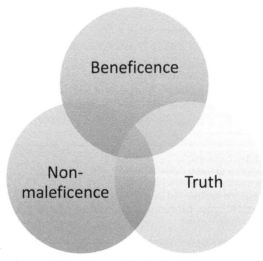

Fig. 1. Ethical issues in surgical training and patient safety.

Box 1
Types of simulation in surgery
• Human cadaver
• Animal cadaver
• Live animal
• Low-fidelity box trainer
• High-fidelity trainer
• Computerized virtual reality

Low-Fidelity Trainers

The introduction of low-fidelity, inanimate simulators, also commonly referred to as *box trainers*, has been met with greater enthusiasm in the surgical training arena. There are several advantages to box trainers (**Box 2**) including the ability to benefit from repetition, that is, "practice makes perfect."

Box trainers are particularly helpful in gaining psychomotor skills related to laparoscopic surgery. Laparoscopy has unique challenges such as adjusting to 2-dimensional judgment of depth and spatial relationships, eye-hand-screen coordination, fulcrum effect of pivoting instruments at varying depths, minimal tissue haptics, amplified tremor, and a reduced surgical field view.[8] Box trainers can recreate these challenges, allowing opportunities for trainees to practice and adjust to these difficulties. Training may be in preparation for clinical experiences or to balance out the lack of a large surgical volume. The value of box trainers in OBGYN training has been shown in randomized study. In 2008, Clevin and Grantcharov[9] randomly assigned OBGYN residents to traditional observing and assisting method versus a structured box trainer laparoscopic simulation program. Not surprisingly, there was significant improvement in the resident group who underwent simulation training in the domains of time, economy of movement, and tissue damage. Similar results by Supe and colleagues[10] were obtained in a larger study and also demonstrated retention of improved skill acquisition at 5 months.

Virtual Reality Simulation

Much attention focuses on the development and use of virtual reality simulators. Computerized virtual reality simulators have been in use in nonmedical fields such as aviation, to improve training and safety.[11] These goals are common to their use in surgical simulation. Virtual reality simulators can offer immediate feedback and often include objective measures for evaluation such as time-motion analysis. The most recent Cochrane Collaborative meta-analysis[12] found that despite acknowledging risk of bias in the studies reviewed, there was evidence in favor of incorporating

Box 2
Advantages of box trainers
• Inexpensive
• Portable
• Unlimited practice
• Provide familiarity with surgical instruments

virtual reality simulation to surgical training programs. Within obstetrics and gynecology, Larsen and colleagues[13] found significant improvement in surgical skills and decreased operating time in residents who were randomly assigned to a virtual reality simulation-based training program compared with standard training for the procedure of laparoscopic salpingectomy. One disadvantage of virtual reality simulators is that their relative cost compared with low-fidelity box trainers is high and, therefore, may not be an option for all interested learners. However, currently, no evidence[12,14] indicates that virtual reality simulators are more effective than low-fidelity box trainers.

CURRENT ROLE OF SIMULATION IN SURGICAL TRAINING

The value of simulation in medical training has been demonstrated by its prevalence in multiple specialties and procedures. Simulation is most prolific and perhaps best formalized in laparoscopy. The Fundamentals of Laparoscopic Skills (FLS) is the first national standardized simulation program in general surgery.[15] Since the introduction of FLS, other specialties, including OBGYN and urology have adopted the program or modification into their own training programs.

Within OBGYN, in the United States, the Accreditation Council for Graduate Medical Education also supports the use of simulation in resident training programs, and the Residency Review Committee recommends that simulation be part of every OBGYN residency training program.[16] In Canada, every OBGYN residency training program has incorporated simulation into their curriculum; however, there is no national standardized simulation curriculum.[17] Despite the lack of a formalized simulation curriculum, there is much enthusiasm for simulation-based training. Simulation has been used to teach a variety of technical skills and procedures in OBGYN (**Box 3**).

Besides providing trainees and surgeons unlimited opportunities to practice a skill or procedure, simulators can provide immediate feedback in a safe environment. The feedback is ideally objective and incorporated into an intentional simulation program. Although rote repetition in simulation increases skill acquisition, the learning curve will plateau without applying the principles of "deliberate practice," as advocated by Ericsson[28] (**Fig. 2**). Others also advocate that learners engage in simulation-based training in a distributed fashion over time,[29,30] as opposed to a single high-intensity and duration exposure. Using these strategies, simulation-based training can be an excellent teaching tool for surgical skills. However, we must be

---

Box 3
Examples of procedure-specific simulation in gynecology

- Loop electrosurgical excision procedure[18]
- Operative hysteroscopy[19]
- Cystoscopy[20]
- Laparoscopic tubal ligation and salpingectomy[21]
- Vaginal hysterectomy[22–24]
- Vaginal repairs[22]
- Total abdominal hysterectomy[25]
- Laparoscopic hysterectomy[26]
- Laparoscopic sacrocolpopexy[27]
- Burch colposuspension[20]

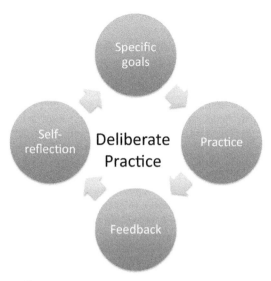

Fig. 2. Deliberate practice.

careful to not assume that a good teaching tool is the same as a good competency assessment tool.

SIMULATION'S ROLE IN COMPETENCY-BASED MEDICAL EDUCATION
Meaning of Competency and Competency-based Medical Education

Traditionally in medicine, a physician is considered competent when he or she is ready to enter independent practice.[31] Many programs have been using outcomes-based education (OBE) in response to the need to ensure trainees are competent at the end of their training. OBE is a method in which program outcomes are emphasized first, and the curriculum processes to obtain these outcomes are secondary (**Fig. 3**). Although OBE aims to train a competent physician by the end of their residency, it is important to consider what being "competent" truly means. The general definition

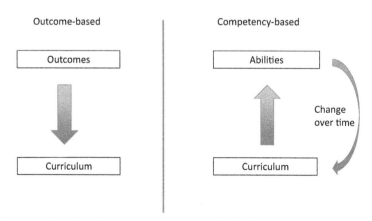

Fig. 3. Outcome-based and competence-based medical education.

is "having the necessary ability of skills" in order "to do something well or well enough to meet a standard."[32]

Competency-based education replaces long lists of learning and knowledge objectives with a curriculum that is organized around abilities. Education organized around long lists of knowledge objectives can result in learning not being integrated into curriculum.[31] An example of this is a trainee having memorized all the risk factors and management options for ectopic pregnancy, but when faced with a real clinical scenario, they struggle to make decisions based on the long list of facts they have committed to memory. A competency-based education model focuses not on the list of facts that must be learned, but strives to design learning experiences that "continuously incorporate prior learning elements and emphasize observable abilities" (see **Fig. 3**).

Competency-based medical education (CBME) views competencies as the ingredients of competence, that is, small elements of learning can be assembled into overarching competency. Additionally, it does not view competency as static. The achievable standard changes from year to year as one transitions through the various levels of training. Even at the completion of education, although an individual may be competent to practice in one setting (such as an academic center), they may find themselves incompetent in another situation (such as a developing country).[31]

Assessment in Competency-based Medical Education

Current assessment techniques in medicine generally rely on proxies to evaluate the trainee (**Table 1**). Examples of this are examinations, assessment of ward activities, and in-training evaluation reports. These techniques often involve indirect observation and little formative assessment. Trainees are often ranked on a Likert scale, which tends to rate all learners above average. Comments about affability are often made rather than descriptions of observable and concrete measures.[33] In contrast, CBME assessments are integrated and longitudinal and rely on multiple objective measures that are aiming to be authentic to the profession. In fact, some would argue CBME assessment is tied to the clinical activities that are thought to define a specialty. Observation occurs "in the trenches" of the clinical setting, rather than a remote experience such as an examination. Evaluation is criterion-based to the specific competency, rather than a normative comparison to other residents.[33]

Adoption of Competency-based Training in North America

Both the Accreditation Council for Graduate Medical Education in the United States and the Royal College of Physicians and Surgeons of Canada have moved toward competency-based system in resident training. The Dutch Society of Obstetricians and Gynecologists has been at the forefront of CBME in our specialty, and their experience in building CBME curriculum can be used by North American programs going forward. At the foundation of the Dutch framework is the idea of an entrustable professional activity (EPA), which is a skill that is observable and measurable and essential

Table 1 Assessment in CBME compared with traditional methods	
Traditional	CBME
• Discrete and summative, often at the end of a program • 5-point Likert-scale normative ranking	• Longitudinal over a training program • Criterion-based to each specific competency • Takes place in the clinical setting

within the specialty. These EPAs are benchmarked across the 6 years of the Dutch training program. Levels are clearly described (**Table 2**) with the standard for each year being clearly defined. For example, basic urogynecology is thought to be something that can be "performed with full supervision–Level 2" at the end of year 2, and "performs without supervision–Level 4" by the end of year 4. In contrast, a lower difficulty task such as uncomplicated antenatal care is benchmarked as "able to supervise others and teach them–Level 5" by end of year 2. As a trainee demonstrates EPAs, they are awarded unsupervised practice in those domains. This technique requires a system of supervision and evaluation by multiple preceptors in the junior years and organized credentialing processes.

Simulation's Role in Achieving Competency

Given the number of factors leading to reduced surgical experience in OBGYN training, it is no surprise that there is already some movement toward using proficiency in simulation as a proxy for surgical competency in the OR. The American Board of Surgery requires demonstrated competency in the Fundamentals of Laparoscopic Surgery as a prerequisite for initial certification.[34] In some centers, the course has even been used for credentialing purposes for practicing surgeons to reduce malpractice insurance rates.[35] Although similar initiatives have not been mandated by OBGYN governing bodies, it is not inconceivable to consider this possibility within this specialty. Given the current climate of increased scrutiny of the profession and attention to patient safety outcomes, despite limited resources, it would be prudent to carefully plan the role of simulation in competency assessment. This is no small undertaking and requires a thorough consideration of limitations and challenges of simulation.

Some critics argue that although simulation can improve knowledge and performance within a simulation environment, there is no evidence that such skill acquisition transfers to performance in the live OR setting. The few studies[21] that attempt to address this concern are weakened by high risk of bias, small numbers, and use of unvalidated measures. However, Gala and colleagues[36] found transfer of skill acquisition in a cohort of 116 OBGYN trainees randomly assigned to control versus faculty-directed sessions in a simulation laboratory using the Fundamentals of Laparoscopic Surgery simulation tasks. The simulation group showed greater improvement using Objective Structured Assessment of Technical Skills[37] in the OR setting as an outcome measure.

Another criticism of surgical simulation includes suboptimal functionality with a limited number of procedures available for simulation. There is also the concern that undue emphasis is placed on technical competencies without defined proficiency-based criteria and equating technical proficiency with procedural competency.

A potential approach to addressing these concerns is viewing the various types of simulation and the skills to be assessed within a hierarchical framework[38] (**Fig. 4**). For

Table 2	
Dutch competency levels	
Level	**Definition**
1	Has knowledge of
2	Performs with full supervision
3	Performs with limited supervision
4	Performs with no supervision
5	Able to supervise others and teach them

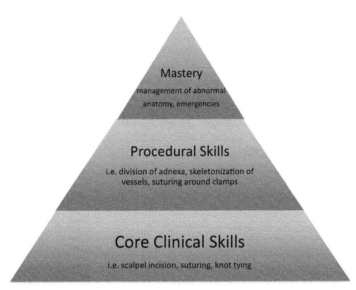

Fig. 4. Hierarchical framework of skills in hysterectomy.

example, if a one considers a total laparoscopic hysterectomy as the procedure of interest, it can be broken down into smaller fragments of skills that build on each other. Core skills include such activities as cutting with a scalpel or scissors, knot tying, cannulating, ligating, aspirating, suturing, cauterizing, retracting, and so on. Low-fidelity simulation materials such as imitation skin, foam, materials from craft stores, or food products, such as tofu or chicken, can be used to mimic human tissue for these activities. Using the Dutch model, level 1 to 2 competency is demonstrated by the ability to perform these skills in an automatic and unconscious manner (**Table 3**). With

Table 3
Dutch levels of competency in laparoscopic hysterectomy

Level	Definition	Laparoscopic Hysterectomy	Simulation
1 2	Has knowledge of Performs with full supervision	• Cutting • Knot tying • Ligating • Suturing • Cauterizing	• Low-fidelity box trainer
3 4	Performs with limited supervision Performs with no supervision	• Laparoscopic entry and closure of ports • Removal or preservation of the adnexa • Skeletonization of the uterine vessels • Possible ureterolysis and closure of the vaginal cuff	• Moderate- to high-fidelity inanimate box trainer • Computerized virtual reality simulation trainer • Cadaveric surgery • Live animal laboratory simulation
5	Able to supervise others and teach them	• Ability to communicate and lead a surgical team (anesthesia, nursing, assists) • Make rapid decisions	• High-fidelity simulation in laboratory with multiple simulated team members

respect to hysterectomy, the next level of competency to be assessed would be procedural skills.

Procedural skills competency depends on the prerequisite of competency in core skills described above and the ability to put these core skills together in a meaningful way to complete a procedure. Examples of procedural skills for total laparoscopic hysterectomy include demonstration of laparoscopic entry and closure of ports, the steps of removal or preservation of the adnexa, skeletonization of the uterine vessels, possible ureterolysis, and closure of the vaginal cuff. In contrast, competency of these procedural skills requires a higher level of knowledge about the relevant pelvic anatomy, pathology, and technical options of instrument choice and handling. This higher level of knowledge allows the operator to modify the usual steps to deal with the multitude of variables encountered in a surgical procedure, such as aberrant anatomy, unexpected bleeding, or equipment malfunction. An inanimate box trainer of moderate to high fidelity or a computerized virtual reality simulator is better suited to assess these procedural competencies, corresponding to Dutch levels 3 to 4. The computerized virtual reality simulator also has the potential advantage of incorporating various anatomic and pathologic features that could contribute to the complexity of a procedure. In our example, the presence of fibroids, adhesions, or endometriosis can increase the complexity of a total laparoscopic hysterectomy.

Simulation can also play a role in evaluating the acquisition of cognitive and nontechnical skills necessary to attain procedural mastery. Procedural mastery encompasses the ability of a surgeon to communicate, make rapid decisions, and lead a surgical team while carrying out a procedure in the OR. This best correlates to the Dutch competency level 5. Simulation aimed specifically at this nontechnical skill set is often neglected in discussions of surgical simulation. However, cognitive skills are an important and perhaps the most sophisticated portion of knowledge necessary for mastery of a procedure and represent the peak of the hierarchical framework. In our example of total laparoscopic hysterectomy, competency assessment requires the roles of anesthesia, nursing, and surgical assists to be simulated in a laboratory setting with the use of a high-fidelity simulator. Although a commercially available model does exist to practice vaginal hysterectomy procedural skills in the Miya model (Miyazaki Enterprises, Winston-Salem, NC), a high-fidelity model for mastery of hysterectomy does not exist. In contrast, a simulator that encompasses procedural skills and demonstration of complex competency does currently exist for obstetrics with the NOELLE (Gaumard Scientific, Miami, FL) or SimMom (Laerdal Medical Canada Ltd, Toronto, ON). If such a model existed for the gynecologic surgical learner, it would require the recreation of variables such as obesity, poor retraction and visualization, pelvic bleeding, and poor tissue quality. The ability of a surgeon to perform a total laparoscopic hysterectomy with technical proficiency while managing a surgical team is a more accurate reflection of competency than perfect scores on a written test or speed on a box trainer. One might also consider it the highest level assessment of simulation-based competency.

TRANSLATION OF SIMULATION COMPETENCY TO SURGICAL COMPETENCY

If the above approach is deemed the best assessment of competency possible using simulation, the next question is whether competency in a simulation setting translates to competency in the OR. Advocates of simulation do not think this type of learning can replace true clinical experience but merely perform it as an adjunct. The worry that simulation experience does not provide real-world skills is related in part to the concern of "decontextualization"[39] of skills in a simulation setting leading to a false

Table 4
Summary of hysterectomy simulator articles

Study	Route	Description	Pros	Cons
Barrier et al,[23] 2012	Vaginal	Low-fidelity model made within a bony resin pelvis of materials widely available	Easily assembled Low per-use cost after initial investment in a resin human pelvis model	No validation No objective evaluation
Greer et al,[24] 2014	Vaginal	Workshop consisting of a low-fidelity model with accompanying lecture and video	Improved resident knowledge and confidence scores	No validation
Geoffrion et al,[22] 2016	Vaginal	Low-fidelity model made of imitation surgical skin and materials found in hardware stores	Established interrater reliability and validity Inexpensive model Evaluates higher levels of competency, such as use of assistants Expert videos accompany model to explain the relevant steps and anatomy	Materials do not approximate human tissue Does not represent vasculature or address adnexa
Tunitsky-Bitton et al,[26] 2016	Laparoscopic	Fundamentals of Laparoscopy trainer and a vaginal cuff constructed with neoprene and swimsuit material	Content and face validity established High interrater reliability	Simulates cuff closure only Requires FLS trainer
King et al,[44] 2015	Laparoscopic	Vaginal cuff made of corduroy and neoprene in a box trainer	Face and content validity and minimum passing score established Low cost ($23) Multiple port sites for surgeon's preference Different materials represent different tissue layers	Simulates cuff closure only

Weizman et al,[45] 2015	Laparoscopic	Latex vaginal cuff in a box trainer	Content and face validity established Recreates the experience of actual needle loading, driving angles, and tissue grasping	Simulates cuff closure only
Hoffman et al,[46] 2012	Robotic	Porcine animal model	Allows practice identifying ovarian vessels and ureters Haptic feedback of tissue manipulation, particularly division of round ligament	Small sample of evaluators High cost ($3000), each animal single use Identification of the cervical vaginal junction difficult, division of paracervical ligaments easier than in humans
Hong et al,[25] 2012	Abdominal	Low-fidelity model assembled from arts and crafts materials	Shown to improve knowledge of anatomy, instruments, and steps of total abdominal hysterectomy Useful for early learner	Nonadaptive Limited use for senior trainees

sense of security regarding an individual's competency. Although previous studies showed that simulation training can improve performance in the OR[12,40] as determined by the Objective Structured Assessment of Technical Skill or Global Rating Scale or speed, the real outcomes of interest are complication rates and OR efficiency. Among the general surgery literature, there is some evidence that simulation training does translate to the OR setting with improved performance and reduction in complications.[41–43] Banks and colleagues[21] reported improved performance in simulation environment and in the OR setting in a small group of trainees randomly assigned to simulation or control. They also suggested that their findings of correlation between the performance scores in the simulation and OR settings provide support for the concept of using simulation performance as a proxy for competency in the OR.

EXISTING SIMULATORS SPECIFIC TO HYSTERECTOMY

Most simulators used in OBGYN and gynecology focus on the acquisition of basic core clinical skills (suturing, knot tying) or laparoscopic models focusing on general procedural skills such as entry, suturing, and port placement. Few simulators exist specifically for hysterectomy, so that procedural skills specific to the procedure and its various routes can be obtained. **Table 4** lists the various hysterectomy simulators that have been published in the literature and their strengths and weaknesses.

As **Table 4** shows, simulation as it exists currently for hysterectomy is limited. Although vaginal hysterectomy has the greatest number of models available, some of which provide experiences such as scalpel use, suturing in deep spaces, and use of assistants, none assess competency beyond the Dutch level 3. Additionally, only 1 simulator is commercially available for training programs to purchase, the Miya Model Vaginal Surgery Training Model (Miyazaki Enterprises, Winston-Salem, NC). This model is a $6500 investment, with replaceable parts, and offers a variety of procedures beyond hysterectomy. It is likely cost prohibitive for many programs, so the contemporary trainee must cobble their simulation experiences together from general clinical skills models and low-fidelity laparoscopic box trainers currently available. In the bigger picture, currently, no one has developed a trainer capable of evaluating the learner in a global operating environment to assess mastery of hysterectomy.

SUMMARY

Simulation in surgery is a valuable teaching tool that has been found to increase skill and knowledge acquisition in trainees. As OBGYN training moves toward a competency-based approach, simulation offers an adjunct to clinical experience. In its present form, simulation offers the best experiences for individuals as they attain early benchmarks of competency. Our general surgery colleagues are already paving the way with programs like FLS, and OBGYN should view this as an inspiration for continuing efforts in developing a standardized simulation curriculum in training programs, and eventually as an adjunct in determining surgical competency.

Areas of Future Study/Development

There is still much work to be done in the areas of well-designed studies to show validity. Future studies should also try to find transferability of skills to the OR. With respect to competency, there will be greater buy-in when simulation-based competency translates into clinically meaningful outcomes such as reduced complication rates and increased efficiency in the OR.

A major reason for slow development of a standardized simulation program in OBGYN is lack of dedicated funding. Funding is not only needed for the actual up-front cost of the simulators but also for the requisite costs of operation and maintenance. These costs can be considered more affordable in the case of low-fidelity box trainers, or, on the other end of the spectrum, prohibitive, in the case of high-fidelity mannequin-type simulators. One such simulator used to teach cesarean sections costs $11,775 (Limbs and Things, Savannah, GA). The robotic virtual reality simulator has a price tag of $100,000 (RoSS, San Jose, CA). There is also the cost associated with on-site instruction by faculty who are not clinically productive during a simulation-based teaching session compared with teaching at the bedside in the OR. Therefore, if any campaign for increased and dedicated funding is going to be successful, all relevant stakeholders need to be involved. This campaign would include not just residency program directors but also the national governing bodies of postgraduate medical education and regulatory licensing bodies when considering competency assessments for certification. In the meantime, the specialty could explore innovative solutions to limitations on faculty time and resources in supporting simulation. For example, our cardiothoracic colleagues have established a Senior Tour,[47] taking advantage of the experience and knowledge of organization of retired surgeons who are able to support simulation training.

OBGYN should consider collaboration with other specialties to advance surgical simulation and capitalize on work already done to increase creativity in addressing challenges. For example, collaboration between the American College of Surgeons and Society of American Gastrointestinal and Endoscopic Surgeons resulted in development and implementation of the Fundamentals of Laparoscopic Surgery.[47]

Another issue that has not been discussed much in the literature is determining the role of industry in development of simulation and credentialing. Much of the recent explosion in new and emerging technologies for surgical application have been funded and often driven by industry. This issue has raised several ethical concerns given the potential conflict of interests. One only has to consider the recent experience with transvaginal mesh to understand this dilemma. However, this conflict of interest is almost unavoidable given the lack of funding in the public sector for the costly endeavors of health care technology research and development. Does this mean that private industry should be responsible for credentialing and certification of new technologies and devices in surgery? Currently, the credentialing process for new technologies has been variable. Sometimes there is a didactic session, sometimes a novice surgeon is proctored by a more experienced surgeon or even a sales representative, and sometimes there is no process at all. It is fair to say that there is increased scrutiny on how such credentialing is taking place, and there may be more enthusiasm for using simulation in this process. Who would be responsible for ensuring the validity of the simulation and transferability to the OR? These questions reinforce that there is need for a transparent and ethical process to address the challenges of how to best adopt rapidly advancing technologies into clinical practice in a cost-effective and safe manner. Simulation could play an important role in this process, but the matter of how it is funded still needs to be negotiated. Credentialing of new technologies is not a small matter and should remain on the agenda going forward.

Up until now, discussions of how simulation can be used to assess competency are only scratching the surface, as they focus almost entirely on technical skills in early stages of training and experience. The future of simulation should move toward assessing procedural mastery, including both technical and nontechnical skills as a summative evaluation for surgeons. Ideally, this assessment will allow the role of simulation to be expanded into the continuing medical education realm to affect surgeons who are already many years into surgical practice.

REFERENCES

1. Education ACfGM. Duty hours in the learning and working environment. Available at: http://www.acgme.org/acgmeweb/tabid/271/GraduateMedicalEducation/DutyHours.aspx. Accessed November 24, 2015.
2. Ontario PAoRi. PARO-CAHO agreement. Available at: http://www.mypraro.ca/Contract/PARO-CAHO_Agreement. Accessed November 24, 2015.
3. Zhan C, Miller MR. Excess length of stay, charges, and mortality attributable to medical injuries during hospitalization. JAMA 2003;290(14):1868–74.
4. Bridges M, Diamond DL. The financial impact of teaching surgical residents in the operating room. Am J Surg 1999;177(1):28–32.
5. Dimitris KD, Taylor BC, Fankhauser RA. Resident work-week regulations: historical review and modern perspectives. J Surg Educ 2008;65(4):290–6.
6. Geoffrion R, Choi JW, Lentz GM. Training surgical residents: the current Canadian perspective. J Surg Educ 2011;68(6):547–59.
7. Graber MA, Wyatt C, Kasparek L, et al. Does simulator training for medical students change patient opinions and attitudes toward medical student procedures in the emergency department? Acad Emerg Med 2005;12(7):635–9.
8. Korndorffer JR Jr, Stefanidis D, Scott DJ. Laparoscopic skills laboratories: current assessment and a call for resident training standards. Am J Surg 2006;191(1):17–22.
9. Clevin L, Grantcharov TP. Does box model training improve surgical dexterity and economy of movement during virtual reality laparoscopy? A randomised trial. Acta Obstet Gynecol Scand 2008;87(1):99–103.
10. Supe A, Prabhu R, Harris I, et al. Structured training on box trainers for first year surgical residents: does it improve retention of laparoscopic skills? A randomized controlled study. J Surg Educ 2012;69(5):624–32.
11. Gaba DM. The future vision of simulation in health care. Qual Saf Health Care 2004;13(Suppl 1):i2–10.
12. Nagendran M, Gurusamy KS, Aggarwal R, et al. Virtual reality training for surgical trainees in laparoscopic surgery. Cochrane Database Syst Rev 2013;(8):CD006575.
13. Larsen CR, Soerensen JL, Grantcharov TP, et al. Effect of virtual reality training on laparoscopic surgery: randomised controlled trial. BMJ 2009;338:b1802.
14. Mulla M, Sharma D, Moghul M, et al. Learning basic laparoscopic skills: a randomized controlled study comparing box trainer, virtual reality simulator, and mental training. J Surg Educ 2012;69(2):190–5.
15. Peters JH, Fried GM, Swanstrom LL, et al. Development and validation of a comprehensive program of education and assessment of the basic fundamentals of laparoscopic surgery. Surgery 2004;135(1):21–7.
16. Education ACfGM. ACGME Program Requirements for Graduate Medical Training in Obstetrics and Gynecology. Available at: http://www.acgme.org/acgmeweb/Portals/0/PFAssets/ProgramRequirements/220_obstetrics_and_gynecology_07012015.pdf. Accessed November 26, 2015.
17. Sanders A, Wilson RD. Simulation training in obstetrics and gynaecology residency programs in Canada. J Obstet Gynaecol Can 2015;37(11):1025–32.
18. Hefler L, Grimm C, Kueronya V, et al. A novel training model for the loop electrosurgical excision procedure: an innovative replica helped workshop participants improve their LEEP. Am J Obstet Gynecol 2012;206(6):535.e1–4.
19. Burchard ER, Lockrow EG, Zahn CM, et al. Simulation training improves resident performance in operative hysteroscopic resection techniques. Am J Obstet Gynecol 2007;197(5):542.e1–4.

20. Fialkow M, Mandel L, VanBlaricom A, et al. A curriculum for Burch colposuspension and diagnostic cystoscopy evaluated by an objective structured assessment of technical skills. Am J Obstet Gynecol 2007;197(5):544.e1–6.
21. Banks EH, Chudnoff S, Karmin I, et al. Does a surgical simulator improve resident operative performance of laparoscopic tubal ligation? Am J Obstet Gynecol 2007;197(5):541.e1–5.
22. Geoffrion R, Suen MW, Koenig NA, et al. Teaching vaginal surgery to junior residents: initial validation of 3 novel procedure-specific low-fidelity models. J Surg Educ 2016;73(1):157–61.
23. Barrier BF, Thompson AB, McCullough MW, et al. A novel and inexpensive vaginal hysterectomy simulator. Simul Healthc 2012;7(6):374–9.
24. Greer JA, Segal S, Salva CR, et al. Development and validation of simulation training for vaginal hysterectomy. J Minim Invasive Gynecol 2014;21(1):74–82.
25. Hong A, Mullin PM, Al-Marayati L, et al. A low-fidelity total abdominal hysterectomy teaching model for obstetrics and gynecology residents. Simul Healthc 2012;7(2):123–6.
26. Tunitsky-Bitton E, Propst K, Muffly T. Development and validation of a laparoscopic hysterectomy cuff closure simulation model for surgical training. Am J Obstet Gynecol 2016;214(3):392.e1–6.
27. Tunitsky-Bitton E, King CR, Ridgeway B, et al. Development and validation of a laparoscopic sacrocolpopexy simulation model for surgical training. J Minim Invasive Gynecol 2014;21(4):612–8.
28. Ericsson KA. Deliberate practice and acquisition of expert performance: a general overview. Acad Emerg Med 2008;15(11):988–94.
29. Mackay S, Morgan P, Datta V, et al. Practice distribution in procedural skills training: a randomized controlled trial. Surg Endosc 2002;16(6):957–61.
30. Moulton CA, Dubrowski A, Macrae H, et al. Teaching surgical skills: what kind of practice makes perfect?: a randomized, controlled trial. Ann Surg 2006;244(3):400–9.
31. Frank JR, Snell LS, Cate OT, et al. Competency-based medical education: theory to practice. Med Teach 2010;32(8):638–45.
32. Merriam-Webster. Merriam-Webster Online Dictionary. Available at: http://www.merriam-webster.com/dictionary/competent. Accessed December 4, 2015.
33. Caccia N, Nakajima A, Scheele F, et al. Competency-Based Medical Education: Developing a Framework for Obstetrics and Gynaecology. J Obstet Gynaecol Can 2015;37(12):1104–12.
34. Surgery ABo. American Board of Surgery Training Requirements. Available at: http://www.absurgery.org/defaul.jsp?certgsque_training. Accessed November 26, 2015.
35. Derevianko AY, Schwaitzberg SD, Tsuda S, et al. Malpractice carrier underwrites Fundamentals of Laparoscopic Surgery training and testing: a benchmark for patient safety. Surg Endosc 2010;24(3):616–23.
36. Gala R, Orejuela F, Gerten K, et al. Effect of validated skills simulation on operating room performance in obstetrics and gynecology residents: a randomized controlled trial. Obstet Gynecol 2013;121(3):578–84.
37. Martin JA, Regehr G, Reznick R, et al. Objective structured assessment of technical skill (OSATS) for surgical residents. Br J Surg 1997;84(2):273–8.
38. Windsor JA. Surgical simulation: what is available and what is needed. Surgeon 2011;9(Suppl 1):S16–8.

39. Brindley PG, Jones DB, Grantcharov T, et al. Canadian Association of University Surgeons' Annual Symposium. Surgical simulation: the solution to safe training or a promise unfulfilled? Can J Surg 2012;55(4):S200–6.

40. Nagendran M, Toon CD, Davidson BR, et al. Laparoscopic surgical box model training for surgical trainees with no prior laparoscopic experience. Cochrane Database Syst Rev 2014;(1):CD010479.

41. Ahlberg G, Enochsson L, Gallagher AG, et al. Proficiency-based virtual reality training significantly reduces the error rate for residents during their first 10 laparoscopic cholecystectomies. Am J Surg 2007;193(6):797–804.

42. Cosman PH, Hugh TJ, Shearer CJ, et al. Skills acquired on virtual reality laparoscopic simulators transfer into the operating room in a blinded, randomised, controlled trial. Stud Health Technol Inform 2007;125:76–81.

43. Seymour NE, Gallagher AG, Roman SA, et al. Virtual reality training improves operating room performance: results of a randomized, double-blinded study. Ann Surg 2002;236(4):458–63 [discussion: 463–4].

44. King CR, Donnellan N, Guido R, et al. Development and Validation of a Laparoscopic Simulation Model for Suturing the Vaginal Cuff. Obstet Gynecol 2015; 126(Suppl 4):27S–35S.

45. Weizman NF, Manoucheri E, Vitonis AF, et al. Design and validation of a novel assessment tool for laparoscopic suturing of the vaginal cuff during hysterectomy. J Surg Educ 2015;72(2):212–9.

46. Hoffman MS. Simulation of robotic hysterectomy utilizing the porcine model. Am J Obstet Gynecol 2012;206(6):523.e1–2.

47. Gardner AK, Scott DJ, Pedowitz RA, et al. Best practices across surgical specialties relating to simulation-based training. Surgery 2015;158(5):1395–402.

Current Issues with Hysterectomy

Matthew A. Barker, MD[a,b,c],*

KEYWORDS

- Hysterectomy • Morcellation • Reimbursement • Quality • Health care reform

KEY POINTS

- Prevalence of leiomyosarcoma in women with uterine fibroids may be overstated.
- Surgical registries may provide clinicians with prospective data to assess risks associated with different types of hysterectomies.
- Reimbursement models are changing to align outcome and quality measures with value.
- Health care reform has led to the correlation of outcome and process measures with reimbursement that may have significant impact on hysterectomy payments in the future.

INTRODUCTION

Hysterectomy is the second most common surgical procedure and the most common gynecologic surgery. One in 9 women will undergo a hysterectomy in their lifetime.[1] The last 30 years witnessed advancements in different types of endoscopic techniques for minimally invasive hysterectomies. The many different techniques offer distinct benefits and risks over the traditional vaginal or abdominal approach. Data to support one route versus another are lacking, especially in relation to robotic-assisted hysterectomy. There has been a strong marketing campaign targeting physicians and hospitals to adopt newer technology despite level 1 evidence of increased costs without benefit.[2] The wide acceptance of other minimally invasive surgical techniques coincided with the launch and use of electric power morcellators. These devices have also been heavily marketed by industry and were adopted widely, despite the absence of safety data.[3]

Technological advancements in surgery must balance safety, quality, costs, and patient engagement. The informed consent process is moving toward patient-centered valuing of surgical risks and benefits and the development of shared decision-making

[a] Department of Obstetrics and Gynecology, Sanford School of Medicine, The University of South Dakota, Vermillion, SD, USA; [b] Department of Internal Medicine, Sanford School of Medicine, The University of South Dakota, Vermillion, SD, USA; [c] Avera McKennan Hospital and University Center, Sioux Falls, SD, USA
* Avera Medical Group-Urogynecology, Plaza 1, 1417 South Cliff Avenue, Suite 101, Sioux Falls, SD 57105.
E-mail address: Matthew.Barker@Avera.org

Obstet Gynecol Clin N Am 43 (2016) 591–601
http://dx.doi.org/10.1016/j.ogc.2016.04.012   **obgyn.theclinics.com**

Abbreviations	
ACO	Accountable Care Organizations
ACOG	American College of Obstetrics and Gynecology
APM	Alternate Payment Model
CMS	Centers for Medicare and Medicaid Services
COEMIG	Center of Excellence in Minimally Invasive Gynecologic Laparoscopists
EHR	Electronic health record
FDA	US Food and Drug Administration
LMS	Leiomyosarcomas
MACRA	Medicare Assess and CHIP (Children's Health Insurance Program) Reauthorization Act of 2015
MIPS	Merit-based Incentive Payment System
MU	Meaningful use
NQF	National Quality Forum
PQRS	The Physician Quality Reporting System
QCDR	Qualified Clinical Data Registry
SGR	Sustainable growth rate
VBPM	Value-based payment modifier

tools and processes for interventions.[4] Growth in patient autonomy has coincided with a reactionary media and political climate that often battles with a medical culture wherein technology is being implemented faster than evidence-based medicine can fully assess all of the risks and benefits. Despite acceptance of minimally invasive hysterectomy techniques, including the use of uterine power morcellation devices, patient perceptions of risk and benefits are often different than their physicians' perceptions. Health care is changing to align physicians, patients, hospitals, and payers to control costs and link reimbursement with improved care, quality, and safety.

The passage of the Medicare Assess and Children's Health Insurance Program Reauthorization Act of 2015 (MACRA) ended the controversial fee-for-service sustainable growth rate (SGR) reimbursement model that had been in place since 1997 and replaced it with reimbursement models based on quality outcome measures and value. What outcome measures are used and how value is defined in performing a hysterectomy should encourage the specialty to focus on the relationship between quality, safety, and cost. It may also allow physicians to compare outcomes of different treatments, control costs, and engage patients in their treatment choices and align their values with their care.

MORCELLATION

The most common indication for hysterectomy is uterine leiomyoma, accounting for an estimated 40% of all hysterectomies performed in the United States.[5] Traditionally, either hysterectomy or myomectomy has been performed through abdominal incisions. Morcellation, a process whereby tissue is divided into smaller pieces so it can be removed from the body, enables surgeons to remove an enlarged uterus or fibroids through scalpel-morcellation vaginally or with mini-laparotomy incisions. As minimally invasive approaches evolved, surgeons first used hand-operated cutting devices to remove the leiomyoma through small laparoscopic incisions. Unfortunately, this technique was hindered by surgeon hand fatigue, development of carpal tunnel and elbow issues in high volume providers, and increased operative times.[6,7] Because of the problems with hand fatigue and longer operative times, the development of an electromechanical-assisted morcellator in 1993 enabled surgeons to now efficiently remove large volumes of tissues efficiently during minimally invasive procedures, leading to a rapid adoption of the procedure. After the introduction of electromechanical-assisted power morcellation, there was a decrease in abdominal hysterectomy rates with 10% of all hysterectomies being done laparoscopically.[8]

Adaptation was made possible because minimally invasive surgical techniques offer an advantage compared with laparotomy. Women undergoing laparoscopic treatment experience fewer wound complications and infections, less blood loss, have decreased risk of deep vein thrombosis, less postoperative pain, shorter hospital stay, and quicker return to normal activity.[9] Ideally, the benefit of minimally invasive hysterectomies and improved efficiencies afforded by electromechanical morcellators should have been balanced with the risk of morcellating an occult malignancy. Although this risk has always been a concern regardless of the mode of hysterectomy, the widespread and untested adaptation of electromechanical morcellation exposed more women to this potential risk.

The American College of Obstetrics and Gynecology (ACOG) developed patient evaluation tools before morcellation to minimize the risk of occult malignancies.[10] These patient evaluation tools include:

1. Negative cervical cytology.
2. Possible pelvic imaging and endometrial assessment depending on clinical presentation.
3. Incidence of uterine cancer and leiomyosarcomas (LMS) with an increase in age, with highest incidence over the age of 65.
4. Postmenopausal women with symptomatic uterine fibroids being at increased risk of an occult malignancy.
5. Uterine size or rapid uterine growth may increase concern for occult malignancy.
6. Women with history of tamoxifen use, history of pelvic radiation, or certain hereditary conditions associated with gynecologic malignancy should not undergo power morcellation.

Unfortunately, preoperative evaluation does not completely eliminate the possibility of an occult malignancy, especially for uterine sarcomas. LMS are rare, occurring in approximately 0.64 per 100,000 women.[11] In fact, there is no presently available test to detect sarcomas before surgery. Consequently, any woman undergoing morcellation needs to understand the unpreventable, yet small risk, of spreading an unrecognized malignancy. This dilemma became national news when a physician underwent morcellation of an unrecognized sarcoma. The couple mounted a media campaign in the national press to draw awareness of the 1 in 400 risk of uterine sarcoma in women undergoing surgery for fibroids.[12] Even though this may be an imprecise estimate of the true incidence of LMS, this event led to a morcellator safety review by the US Food and Drug Administration (FDA). During this investigation, the FDA concluded that 1 in 350 women undergoing hysterectomy or myomectomy for the treatment of fibroids will have an unsuspected uterine LMS.[13,14] Power morcellators posed an unacceptably high risk of spreading cancer, and consequently, the FDA released a black box warning in 2014 discouraging its use.[14] This opinion has had a chilling effect in the minimally invasive gynecologic surgery community and resulted in near worldwide suspension of sales of the device.

Since this announcement, there have been several publications that question the incidence of LMS reported by the FDA. If non-peered-reviewed studies and atypical leiomyoma were excluded, there were only 8 cases of LMS among 12,402 women having surgery for presumed leiomyoma: a prevalence of 1 in 1550 or 0.064%.[7] A recent meta-analysis of 133 studies report similar prevalence of LMS among women undergoing fibroid surgery (1 in 1960 or 0.051%).[15] In a large population-based prospective registry study, the reported prevalence of LMS was only 2 of 8720 (0.023%), although the overall rate of uterine malignancy was 0.13%, in women undergoing laparoscopic supracervical hysterectomies.[16] In a statewide quality and safety database of women undergoing benign hysterectomies, the incidence of unexpected gynecologic malignancy was 2.7%, although the rate of sarcoma was 0.22%.[17] In an open letter to the FDA, many leaders in the gynecologic surgery community criticized the FDA's conclusions and called for modification of the FDA's current restrictive guidance regarding power morcellation.[18]

Clinical recommendations suggested the following[18]:

1. Risk of leiomyosarcoma is higher in the older population; greater caution should be exercised before recommending morcellation procedure for these patients.
2. Women age 35 years and older with irregular uterine bleeding and presumed fibroids should have an endometrial biopsy and normal results of cervical cancer screening.
3. Ultrasound or MRI findings of large irregular vascular mass, often with irregular anechoic (cystic) areas reflecting necrosis, may cause suspicion for LMS.
4. Women wishing minimally invasive procedures with morcellation, including scalpel morcellation either abdominally or vaginally, or power morcellation using laparoscopic guidance, should understand potential risk of decreased survival may LMS be present. Open procedures should be offered to all women considering minimally invasive procedures for fibroids.
5. Following morcellation, careful inspection for tissue fragments should be undertaken and copious irrigation of the pelvic and abdominal cavities should be performed to minimize risk of retained tissue.

The controversy following the FDA communication focused the attention of gynecologic surgeons on the risks and benefits of morcellation. Although all techniques for debulking the uterus carry the risk of spreading occult malignancies, the prevalence of LMS appears to be exceeding low. Moreover, to factor only the impact of upstaging occult malignancies potentially obscures the overall risks associated with a return to laparotomy. In a survey of minimally invasive gynecologic surgeons' responses to the FDA safety communication, 45% had to stop using power morcellation due to hospital mandate, and 45% reported an increase in their rate of laparotomy.[19] In the same survey, more than 80% of respondents thought that the communication has not led to improvement in patient outcomes.[19] More importantly, in a decision analysis study, Siedhoff and colleagues[20] compared 100,000 hypothetical women having laparoscopic hysterectomy with 100,000 having open hysterectomy for presumed leiomyomata. Even though there were more deaths from LMS in the laparoscopic surgical group, overall mortality was lower compared with the laparotomy group because of fewer perioperative deaths, pulmonary or venous emboli, and wound infections. When hysterectomies were compared the year before and after the 2014 FDA communication, there was a decrease in laparoscopic hysterectomies and an increase in abdominal and vaginal hysterectomies.[21] There was also an increase in major complications and 30-day hospital readmission rates.[21]

ACOG recommended the FDA establish a national, prospective morcellation surgery registry to acquire an adequate volume of consistent and reliable data.[10] Until more data are available, surgeons using power morcellator should perform the procedure in the confines of a bag to minimize the risk of unexpected seeding of undiagnosed malignancies. Further research is needed to allow clinicians to better differentiate leiomyoma from sarcomas before surgery. The surgeon should provide a thorough review of the nuanced risk-benefit ratio for leiomyoma morcellation to better inform the patient during the informed consent process before undergoing hysterectomy or myomectomy.

REIMBURSEMENT AND HEALTH CARE REFORM

As alternative payment models are developed, such as accountable care organizations (ACO) or bundled payments, and as other areas of medicine implement pay for performance, hysterectomy payments may soon be based on a physician's adherence to processes or to individual outcomes.[22] Reporting outcomes related to hysterectomy is complicated. Nevertheless, given how common the procedure is, patients deserve confirmation that this procedure is done at a certain level of quality and safety, and that costs are controlled.

Gynecologists have been at the forefront of innovation to make hysterectomies safer and less invasive with shorter recovery for patients, but government payers and regulations are starting to influence practice patterns. How obstetricians and gynecologists are paid will dramatically change in 2019. The passage of MACRA in 2015 replaces the SGR reimbursement model that had been in place since 1997, incentivizes providers to adopt alternative payment models, and combines existing quality reporting programs into one new system.[23] In 2019, the traditional financial incentives for the fee-for-service volume model will be phased out and replaced with models that will adjust payment either negatively or positively based on quality outcome measures and value.[23]

Physicians will have the choice of enrolling in 2 types of payment plans, or opt-out completely. A physician may choose to participate in either an alternate payment model (APM) or the merit-based incentive payment system (MIPS).

Merit-based Incentive Payment System

The Physician Quality Reporting System (PQRS), Meaningful Use (MU), and Value-Based Payment Modifier (VBPM) will be transitioned into MIPS after 2018. Practices that are already participating in all or some of these programs will find transitioning into MIPS easier because this program has elements of all these programs. Payment will be based on value instead of volume. The definition of value is not clear and up for debate, but at its core will be a function of quality, health information technology, resource use, and clinical practice improvement. Payment bonuses or penalties will be based on a 100-point MIPS composite performance score in which providers are evaluated in 4 categories. The performance threshold will be set annually and known to physicians before the start of each year.[24]

Quality (30 points)

PQRS will continue through 2018, but the data collected in 2017 will be the first year to report quality measures that will affect payments under MIPS in 2019. Only 6 of the 280 measures now available through PQRS reporting deal with preoperative evaluation or offer surgical alternatives to patients. None of these are unique to gynecology. The American Taxpayer Relief Act of 2014 mandated the development of alternative PQRS reporting pathways. This new pathway will allow individuals and group practices to submit data through a qualified clinical data registry (QCDR) instead of claims-based reporting of PQRS measures. QCDR measures will have to prove to be worthy of measurement over time, or they will be eliminated.

Currently, Centers for Medicare and Medicaid Services (CMS) requires 9 specialty-specific measures to be reported, although up to 30 can be included in a QCDR and reported. ACOG has recommended registries for robotic surgery and morcellator use to assess safety, but these measures have to prove worthy of measurement over time and translate into better patient outcomes for it to be associated with MIPS.[10,25]

QCDRs have to be approved through a formal process before one can use them as PQRS.

Meaningful use of technology (25 points)

Practices that have implemented MU (either stage 1 or stage 2) using a certified electronic health record (EHR) will have met this component of MIPS because it will be required in this payment system. Capturing outcome measures and streamlining the EHR to report data easily will be important to workflows for practices. Outcome measures that may need to be reported as it relates to hysterectomies in the future may include capturing readmission data and/or capturing the right diagnosis or procedural codes.

Resource use (30 points)

The VBPM program was set up to reimburse based on quality and cost, thus designed to be a measure of resource use. Practices that participate in PQRS have had payments adjusted up, down, or the same depending on where they fell in relation to the mean, using a combination of claims to measure cost and PQRS to measure quality. The goal of the system is to adjust based on risk, such that, the sicker the patient a practice manages the system considers this so as to not automatically penalize the practice. Reporting and clearly capturing comorbidities that patients have who had a hysterectomy could become vital to avoiding penalties. It will also encourage physicians and hospitals to integrate and coordinate clinical services before admission, during hospital stay, and after discharge to control costs.

Clinical practice improvement (15 points)

This component is new for 2019 and will require physicians to follow their outcome and show that they are improving care. Physicians will get credit for their clinical quality improvement activities as well as transitioning to the patient-centered medical home or the patient-centered medical home specialty practice model. Components of practice improvement may include population management, care coordination, expanded practice access, or patient safety and practice assessment. Coordinating care in areas that have limited access to obstetricians and gynecologists may be a component of this or coordinating gynecologic services for specific health conditions. Coordinating hysterectomy management and follow-up may count toward practice improvement. Also, practice changes that seek to reduce readmissions or reduce costs associated with hysterectomy may also count.

Alternate Payment Model

The goal of APM is to incentivize quality and value. Examples of this could include ACOs, patient-centered medical homes, bundled payments, warrantied surgeries, and condition-based payments. In bundled payments, a single payment could be made to 2 or more providers who are currently paid separately (eg, hospital + physician). With warrantied surgeries, there would be a higher payment for quality of care and no extra payment for complications or preventable errors during a specified period. In condition-based payments, payment is specific for the condition, not for procedures or other care delivered. The goal of all these systems is to decrease unnecessary procedures and reward positive quality outcomes. CMS has already started some of these models, such as ACOs or the patient-centered medical home. Additional new models will be developed later. For an eligible provider to receive bonus payments through these models, they must meet certain thresholds. An APM must use certified EHR technology and provide payment based on quality measures and either bare "more than nominal" financial risk for monetary losses or be a medical home model. Physicians will have to meet certain thresholds to be "qualified participants" and qualify for incentive payments, which will be phased in over time. In 2019, 25% of Medicare revenue must be in APM, and this will increase to 75% by 2023. In the future, there may be APMs for specific gynecologic diseases or procedures like hysterectomies that will bonus practices that keep costs down. This incentive to decrease cost may have a greater influence on the route of hysterectomy performed and resources used to perform the procedure to contain cost and decrease complications. Examples of this already exist with total joint replacements in orthopedics and in cardiac surgery.[26]

In 2016, CMS launched the Comprehensive Care for Joint Replacement model, which will hold hospitals accountable for the quality of care they deliver to Medicare fee-for-service beneficiaries for hip and knee replacements from surgery through recovery.[27] The goal of this program is to provide hospitals a financial incentive to work with physicians, home health agencies, skilled nursing homes, and other providers to coordinate care. Hospitals will be reimbursed a standard amount for each surgery, and this standard bundled reimbursement will cover all these costs. Any failure to meet certain standards will lead to the hospital being penalized and not receiving the full payment, but the hospital may be penalized if it is not able to coordinate care and contain costs. Across the United States, bundled payments are not only being trialed through government mandates, but also private payers are considering this method of reimbursement to control costs. Private payers are already trying to control costs in regards to hysterectomy by eliminating prior authorization if hysterectomy is planned to be performed by the vaginal route. Given the decreased costs of vaginal hysterectomy compared with other minimally invasive and abdominal routes of hysterectomy, payers may be looking at working with hospitals to use bundled payments as a way to influence surgeons into performing safer and less expensive surgery. Government and private payers look at this type of influence as encouraging care coordination and linking payments with surgical outcomes.

MACRA ends SGR, and providers will see a 0.5% annual increase in reimbursement through 2019. However, those rates will freeze from 2020 to 2025. Those providers who participate in APM and are exempt from MIPS will receive an annual lump-sum bonus payment of 5% of their prior-year covered Medicare Part B professional payments during 2019 through 2024. Higher annual reimbursement rates increase after 2025, but merit-based payments are subject to positive or negative performance adjustments. In 2019, the maximum bonus will be ±4%, but will grow to ±9% in 2022 and beyond for providers enrolled in MIPS. However, MIPS adjustments will be budget neutral.[23] Per the MACRA law, quarterly reports are to be furnished to physicians during the year so that they can monitor their progress. Those who chose to opt out of MIPS or APM, or who are not eligible, will see lower reimbursement rates after 2025. Physicians will continue to bill in the traditional fee-for-service manner, but process and quality metrics may be attached to these codes, affecting the overall bonus and reimbursement. Physicians who try APMs, but do not meet the necessary quality and revenue thresholds, will revert to an evaluation under the MIPS model. It is up to many of the specialty societies to develop models and quality metrics for consideration by the Department of Health and Human Services for use in MIPS and APMs.[28]

The largest change that obstetricians and gynecologists will see from MACRA and CMS is the development of quality metrics and outcome measures specific to specialties. The National Quality Forum (NQF) is a contracted vendor that reviews and endorses measures based on their clinical importance, performance gap, and their validity and reliability. The NQF has rigorous standards that may take years to approve a measure. It is expected that CMS will be more likely to accept future measures for PQRS with NQF endorsement.[29,30] NQF does not create measures. Rather, measures need to be developed by other organizations (including Agency for Healthcare Research and Quality, health care systems, and quality collaborative), field tested, and validated before submission. CMS and the America's Health Insurance Plans recently announced plans to work with the NQF, medical specialty societies, employer groups, and consumer groups under an umbrella organization called the Core Quality Measures Collaborative to derive a set of measures that are meaningful to patients, consumers, and physicians, while reducing variability in measure selection, collection burden, and costs. The measure sets will be implemented and updated through the physician fee schedule in MIPS and APMs. Private payers are expected to implement these quality measures as physician contracts come up for renewal.

Currently, the quality measures recognized by NQF related to benign hysterectomies include performing cystoscopy at the time of hysterectomy for pelvic organ prolapse to detect lower urinary tract injury.[30] Recently, endorsed quality measures now include performing a vaginal apical suspension at the time of hysterectomy to address pelvic organ prolapse and preoperative evaluation for stress urinary incontinence before hysterectomy for pelvic organ prolapse.[30] These measures are considered process measures that are self-reported and obtained from the EHR. Some of these future measures will rely on specialty QCDR registries for reports. CMS updates information on measures and reporting frequently.[23,31]

The NQF does recognize areas of gaps and concepts for which measures might provide important contributions to outcomes, including assessing functional status related to urinary incontinence following hysterectomy. Surgery outcomes measures address management of symptomatic uterine leiomyoma, disorders of menstrual bleeding, and when to appropriately use power morcellation in gynecologic surgery. Given the controversy with morcellation, this may create a process whereby gynecologists devise practice patterns and standard processes for physicians to follow and collect data on all patients using the device as opposed to only those with complications. The only other currently NQF-endorsed gynecologic-specific measured benchmark is making sure endometrial sampling has been performed before endometrial ablation.[30] Using registries and standardized reporting mechanisms may help assess safety and quality of new devices and procedures. Individual specialty organizations are already submitting registries to CMS for QCDR approval, such as the American Urogynecologic Society and their Pelvic Floor Disorders Registry. The American Association of Gynecologic Laparoscopists created a Center of Excellence in Minimally Invasive Gynecologic Laparoscopists (COEMIG). There are no data to support the benefits of COEMIG certification, but it does provide standard requirements for surgeons and facilities to perform minimally invasive gynecologic procedures as well as surgical outcome data that can be used for quality assurance and improvement.[24] Centers of Excellence may enable providers to meet the multiple components of MIPS, including practice improvement, tracking process, and outcome measures, but there is often an initiation and annual membership fee. Physicians should be looking at developing coordinated care processes that will help them be successful at meeting process and outcome measures being developed by CMS, payers, and medical societies. Physician's ability to work with payers, hospitals, and their colleagues to coordinate safe and efficient care for women requiring hysterectomies will be key to the transition to alternative payment models.

DISCUSSION

Health care reform will have a profound impact on gynecologists who see Medicare beneficiaries. Despite this patient population being a small percentage of the patients in obstetrics and gynecology, the changes to reimbursements have the potential to greatly influence Medicaid and private payers. It will also change how care is coordinated and will drive future reporting on quality and performance metrics. Payers will be looking at which process, outcome, and quality metric lead to better and more cost-efficient care.

As the focus changes to reporting outcome measures, medical societies and payers must work toward approving evidence-based and relevant quality measures. Controversy exists regarding whether quality metrics should be process measures (eg, reporting how many patients get the recommended preoperative antibiotics) or outcomes measures (eg, the proportion of patients with surgical infection).[24] The latter focuses on patient-centered outcomes rather than a proxy metric, but physicians may prefer process measures to avoid being penalized for caring for higher-risk patients. Given the potential media backlash from complications arising from surgical therapy, our goal should be to restore trust and faith in the medical system by promoting care that decreases risk and promotes value. Rather than criticize federal organizations for failures in analyzing retrospective data on new therapies, physicians should support processes that prospectively track new technology for safety and quality and control its application and utilization. Well-designed and implemented registries may become the new pathway for innovative change in the hysterectomy procedure. Value will be found when physicians, payers, and patients are equally engaged and committed to a system that aligns quality, safety, and costs.

REFERENCES

1. Wu JM, Wechter ME, Geller EJ, et al. Hysterectomy rates in the United States, 2003. Obstet Gynecol 2007;110:1091–5.
2. Moen M, Walter A, Harmanli O, et al. Considerations to improve the evidence-based use of vaginal hysterectomy in benign gynecology. Obstet Gynecol 2014;124:585–8.
3. Nygaard I. Balancing innovation and harm. Am J Obstet Gynecol 2014;210:383–4.
4. Weinstein JN, Clay K, Morgan TS. Informed patient choice: patient-centered valuing of surgical risks and benefits. Health Aff (Millwood) 2007;26:726–30.
5. Whiteman MK, Hillis SD, Jamieson DJ, et al. Inpatient hysterectomy surveillance in the United States, 2000-2004. Am J Obstet Gynecol 2008;198:34.e1–7.
6. Carter JE, McCarus SD. Laparoscopic myomectomy: time and cost analysis of power versus manual morcellation. J Reprod Med 1997;42:383–8.
7. Parker WH, Pritts EA, Olive DL. What is the future of open intraperitoneal power-morcellation of fibroids? Clin Obstet Gynecol 2016;159:73–84.
8. Farquhar CM, Steiner CA. Hysterectomy rates in the United States 1990-1997. Obstet Gynecol 2002;99:229–34.
9. Aarts JWM, Nieboer TE, Johnson N, et al. Surgical approach to hysterectomy for benign gynecologic disease. Cochrane Database Syst Rev 2015;(8):CD003677.
10. Power morcellation and occult malignancy in gynecologic surgery. Washington, DC: American College of Obstetricians and Gynecologists; 2014. Available at: www.ACOG.org.
11. Zivanovic O, Leitao MM, Iasonos A, et al. Stage-specific outcomes of patients with uterine leiomyosarcoma: a comparison of the International Federation of Gynecology and Obstetrics and American Joint Committee on Cancer Staging Systems. J Clin Oncol 2009;27:2066–72.

12. Women's health alert: deadly cancers of the uterus spread by gynecologists. Stop morcellating the uterus in minimally invasive and robot assisted hysterectomy and myomectomy. Change.org Inc. Available at: https://www.change.org/p/women-s-health-alert-deadly-cancers-of-the-uterus-spread-by-gynecologists-stop-morcellating-the-uterus-in-minimally-invasive-and-robot-assisted-hysterectomy. Accessed February 27, 2016.

13. Laparoscopic uterine power morcellation in hysterectomy and myomectomy: FDA safety communication. Available at: http://www.fda.gov/MedicalDevices/Safety/AlertsandNotices/ucm393576.htm. Accessed February 6, 2016.

14. Laparoscopic uterine power morcellation in hysterectomy and myomectomy: FDA safety communication. Available at: http://www.fda.gov/MedicalDevicesSafety/AlertsandNotices/ucm42443.htm. Accessed February 6, 2016.

15. Pritts E, Vanness D, Berek J, et al. The prevalence of occult leiomyosarcoma at surgery for presumed uterine fibroids: a meta-analysis. Gynecol Surg 2015; 12(3):165–77.

16. Bojahr B, De Wilde R, Tchartchian G. Malignancy rate of 10,731 uteri morcellated during laparoscopic supracervical hysterectomy (LASH). Arch Gynecol Obstet 2015;292:665–72.

17. Mahnert N, Morgan D, Campbell D, et al. Unexpected gynecologic malignancy diagnosed after hysterectomy performed for benign indications. Obstet Gynecol 2015;125:397–405.

18. Parker W, Berek JS, Pritts E, et al. An open letter to the FDA regarding the use of morcellation procedures for women having surgery for presumed uterine fibroids. J Minim Invasive Gynecol 2016;23(3):303–8.

19. Lum DA, Sokol ER, Berek JS, et al. FDA warnings against power morcellation. J Minim Invasive Gynecol 2016. http://dx.doi.org/10.1016/j.jmig2016.01.019.

20. Siedhoff MT, Wheeler SB, Rutstein SE, et al. Laparoscopic hysterectomy with morcellation vs abdominal hysterectomy for presumed fibroid tumors in premenopausal women: a decision analysis. Am J Obstet Gynecol 2015;212:591.e1-8.

21. Harris JA, Swenson CW, Uppal S, et al. Practice patterns and postoperative complications before and after US Food and Drug Administration safety communication on power morcellation. Am J Obstet Gynecol 2016;214:98.e1–13.

22. Gaba ND, Polite FG, Keller JM, et al. To err is human; to provide safe, quality, and cost-effective hysterectomy is divine! Clin Obstet Gynecol 2014;57:128–39.

23. Centers for Medicare & Medicaid Services, Physician Quality Reporting System 2016. Available at: https://www.cms.gov/Medicare/Quality-Initiatives-Patient-Assessment-Instruments/PQRS/Registry-Reporting.html. Accessed February 29, 2016.

24. Cadish LA, Richardson EE. The end of the Medicare sustainable growth rate. Obstet Gynecol 2015;126:613–6.

25. Robotic Surgery in Gynecology. ACOG committee opinion No. 628. American College of Obstetricians and Gynecologists. Obstet Gynecol 2015;125:760–7.

26. Rosenman AE. AUGS 36th presidential address: "The Journey of a Thousand Miles Begins with a Single Step" (Lao Tzu). Female Pelvic Med Reconstr Surg 2016;22:3–6.

27. United States, Department of Health and Human Services, Centers for Medicare & Medicaid Services, "Comprehensive Care for Joint Replacement Model," Fact Sheet. 2015. Available at: https://innovation.cms.gov/initiatives/cjr. Accessed February 28, 2016.

28. Congressional Budget Office, "re: Cost Estimate and Supplemental Analyses for H.R. 2, the Medicare Access and CHIP Reauthorization Act 2015", March 25, 2015.

29. Hale DS. Pay for performance—are you prepared? Female Pelvic Med Reconstr Surg 2016;22(3):123–5.
30. NQF-Endorsed Measures for Surgical Procedures. 2015. Available at: http://www. qualityforum.org/Publications/2015/12/Surgery_2014_Final_Report.aspx. Accessed February 28, 2016.
31. CMS and major commercial health plans, in concert with physician groups and other stakeholders, announce alignment and simplification of quality measures. Available at: https://www.cms.gov/Medicare/Quality-Initiatives-Patient-Assessment-Instruments/QualityMeasures/Core-Measures.html. Accessed February 28, 2016.

Index

Note: Page numbers of article titles are in **boldface** type.

Obstet Gynecol Clin N Am 43 (2016) 603–609
http://dx.doi.org/10.1016/S0889-8545(16)30052-3
0889-8545/16/$ – see front matter

obgyn.theclinics.com

Moving?

Make sure your subscription moves with you!

To notify us of your new address, find your **Clinics Account Number** (located on your mailing label above your name), and contact customer service at:

Email: journalscustomerservice-usa@elsevier.com

800-654-2452 (subscribers in the U.S. & Canada)
314-447-8871 (subscribers outside of the U.S. & Canada)

Fax number: 314-447-8029

Elsevier Health Sciences Division
Subscription Customer Service
3251 Riverport Lane
Maryland Heights, MO 63043

ELSEVIER

Printed and bound by CPI Group (UK) Ltd, Croydon, CR0 4YY

07/10/2024

01040504-0003